One Bite at a Time

D0730971

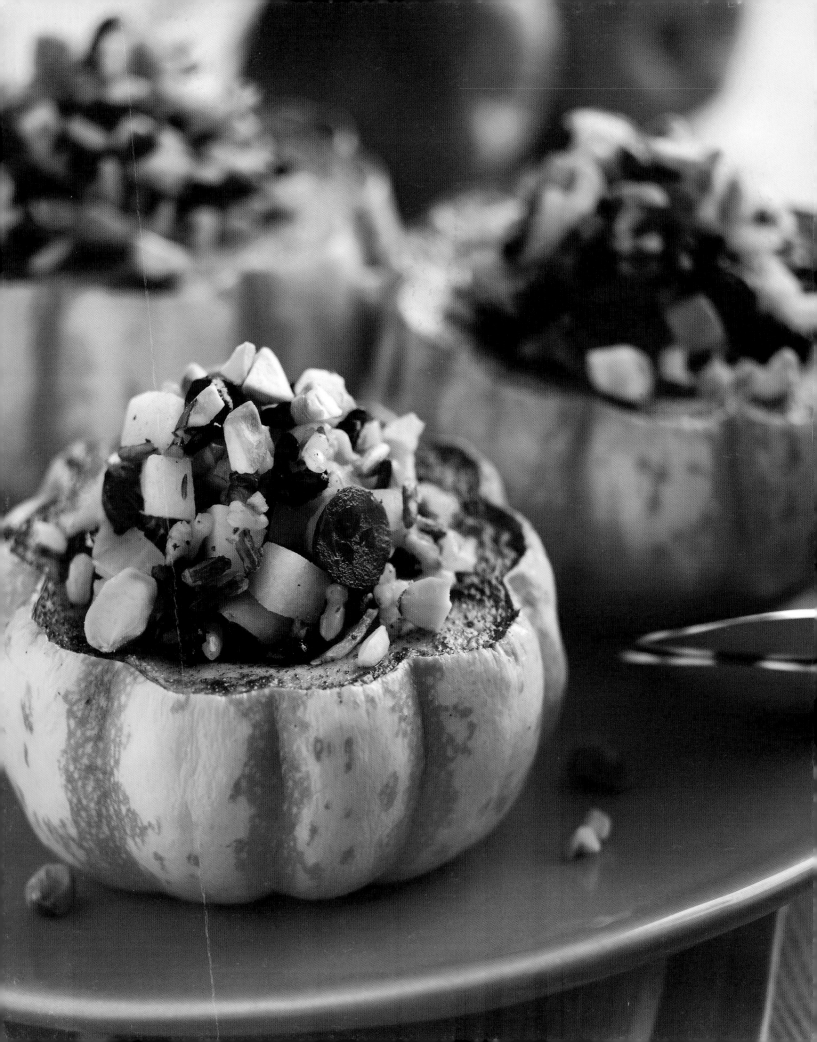

One Bite at a Time

Nourishing Recipes for Cancer Survivors
and Their Friends

Second Edition

Rebecca Katz
with Mat Edelson

CELESTIAL ARTS
Berkeley | Toronto

Celestial Arts
an imprint of Ten Speed Press
PO Box 7123
Berkeley, California 94707
www.tenspeed.com

Distributed in Australia by Simon & Schuster Australia, in Canada by Ten Speed Press Canada, in New Zealand by Southern Publishers Group, in South Africa by Real Books, and in the United Kingdom and Europe by Publishers Group UK.

Cover design by Nancy Austin
Book design by Leslie Harrington and Chloe Rawlins
Photographs on page 147 by Rebecca Katz
Photographs on pages 1, 125, 129, 133, 139, 147, and 149 by Lori Eanes
Food styling by Karen Shinto
Food styling assistance by Katie Christ
Prop styling by Emma Star Jensen

Library of Congress Cataloging-in-Publication Data

Katz, Rebecca.
  One bite at a time: nourishing recipes for cancer survivors and their friends / Rebecca Katz with Mat Edelson. — 2nd ed.
      p. cm.
  Includes index.
  Summary: "A cookbook for cancer patients with more than 85 recipes, featuring full nutritional analysis and anecdotes from cancer survivors"—Provided by publisher.
  ISBN 978-1-58761-327-2 (pbk.) — ISBN 978-1-58761-333-3 (cloth)
  1. Cancer—Diet therapy—Recipes. I. Edelson, Mat. II. Title.

RC271.D52K38 2008
641.5'631—dc22

2008013427

Printed in China
First printing this edition, 2008
1 2 3 4 5 6 7 8 9 10 - 12 11 10 09 08

Dedication
For my parents

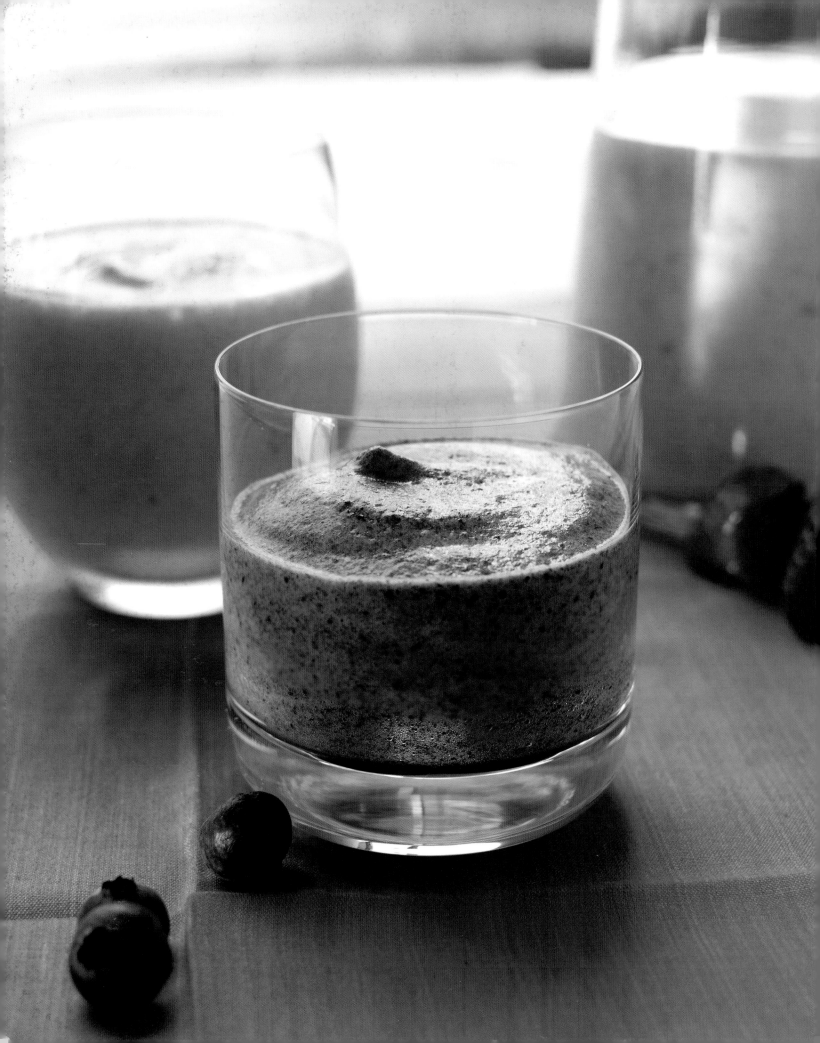

Contents

Foreword

Sometimes a little blessing drops in your lap when you least expect it. When I was asked to look at the manuscript for this book, I have to admit to feeling paradoxically both grateful and ambivalent. Grateful because, as both a colorectal cancer survivor and a patient educator, the subject of eating well, and especially tastefully, while living with cancer is a topic most doctors do not address.

OVERWHELMED PATIENTS DO NOT THINK TO ASK ABOUT EATING WELL. At the very least, I felt that a book such as this one would give medical professionals something to hand to patients. And yet, this was the source of my ambivalence as well, for the very few cookbooks aimed at cancer patients that have been published (many of which sit on my office shelf) just don't grab you by the taste buds. These books tend to take a utilitarian approach to eating, with taste weighing in as a secondary factor.

And then there is this little gem. A little voice kept going off in my head as I read through the recipes and the accompanying text. It kept saying "yes, yes. Yes!!!" That was the voice of the survivor in me speaking. In tone, content, and taste, it is clear that chef Rebecca Katz really is a kindred spirit who doesn't approach her work clinically, but rather from the heart. And yet (and I suppose this appeals to the educator in me) she approaches this book as a consummate professional.

If Rebecca were just an ordinary caring chef, that in itself would be appreciated. It is obvious that she delights in creating delicious recipes. However, it is abundantly apparent that Rebecca approaches this book with a depth of understanding for a survivor's needs that, quite honestly, I've never before seen in a chef.

Her recipes combine taste with powerful immune-building ingredients, which are always at the forefront of a survivor's mind. I know that having had cancer once makes me statistically more vulnerable to a relapse, so I want to eat foods that are rich in cancer-fighting antioxidants and vitamins.

Perhaps most impressive is Rebecca's knowledge of how a survivor's appetite changes while moving through the different phases of cancer diagnosis, treatment, recovery, and survivorship.

At every step, Rebecca is a true educator herself, informing survivors and their loved ones how to ride out the emotional and physiological roller coaster while staying tastefully nourished.

Speaking from personal experience, one of the most difficult aspects for a cancer patient is the unpredictability of one's appetite from one day to the next especially during cancer treatments. This book takes that frustration away. It does the explaining for you. If you're not up to cooking yourself, this book gently teaches friends and family how to prepare and bring over a wide variety of small meals that store well and are certain to offer options to fit varying appetites. That's so important for everyone's morale. Nothing makes my patients sadder during treatment than when their wonderful friends bring over foods they cannot (or should not) eat. Obviously this is no one's "fault" as everyone is just playing it by ear. No more. This book takes away the guesswork, which is why I'm making sure each of my patients gets a copy. Now, when their caregivers ask "is there something I can make for you?" they can hand them this book and say "anything in here would be great!" Truthfully, I only wish I'd had this book when I was sick.

Regardless of where you are on your cancer journey, you'll find something incredibly useful and uplifting within these pages. In some ways this is far more than a cookbook. It's like sitting down with a compassionate friend.

Rebecca gets it.

Her down-to-earth tone is that of a close confidant, her words flavored with a savvy and wisdom that only come from personal experience. I'm glad she's now a part of my life. After you read and use this book, I'm sure you'll feel the same way.

—Eden Stotsky, MSEd

Director, Patient Education
Johns Hopkins Colon Cancer Center

Acknowledgments

This book was conceived and brought to life with the help of a wonderfully supportive community.

MY THANKS AND GRATITUDE GO TO THE FOLLOWING PEOPLE FOR HELP IN CREATING THE FIRST EDITION OF THIS BOOK: Eden Stotsky, MSEd, cancer survivor and Director of Patient Education, Johns Hopkins Colon Cancer Center, for her lovely foreword and support of this project; Marsha Tomassi, for her tremendous contribution of time and energy; Chet Grycz, for opening the door to Celestial Arts; Linda Hawkins, recipe tester, and the only person who actually got me to use a measuring spoon—your patience and tenacity enhanced the recipes in this book; and to the community of volunteers who tested recipes for the first edition, and provided invaluable feedback. My thanks also go to the Ten Speed/Celestial Arts team who helped make the first edition a reality: Jo Ann Deck, who saw the possibility of what could be—you are the ultimate fairy godmother; Lorena Jones for her clarity and vision; Carrie Rodrigues, project editor; Lisa Regul for her publicity expertise; Leslie Harrington, Nancy Austin, and Chloe Rawlins for the sensitivity of the book's design; and Scott Peterson and his team—Jason Drescher, Karen Shinto, Katie Christ, and Emma Star Jensen—for the beautiful photography.

Thanks also go to Gary Bang; Shannon McGowan, her daughter Liz Behrens, son John Behrens, and sister Susan Dyer; Andrea Riesenfeld; Jennifer Omholt; Aliyah Stein and daughter Lailah Roberston, for their inspirational and courageous stories; Paula Bartholomy, co-founder and director of Hawthorn University; Sarah Bearden and Donna Shoemaker for freely sharing their expertise and enthusiasm in the area of nutrition; Daniel L. Junck, MD, friend and colleague, for the knowledge and humor that you brought to our Culinary Solutions for Health and Healing workshops; and Nathan Boone, for your guidance and advice on organic farming.

Many thanks to the following people for their invaluable contributions to the second edition: my agent, Jeremy Katz, for his belief in my work, and for keeping me pointed in the right direction; Melissa Moore, my editor at Ten Speed/Celestial Arts for her guidance, compassion, and editorial flair, which have made this second edition even better than I could have imagined; Wendy Remer, gifted baker and extraordinary chocolatier, for her expertise in reformulating some of the baked good recipes; photographer Lori Eanes for spending a day in my kitchen shooting the "fantasy pantry" and for her other photographic contributions; Wendy Hess, for the newly added nutritional analysis accompanying each recipe, and the daily weather reports from Vermont; Jodie Chase, for getting me and this book out into the world; Karen Omholt and Linda Dalton for their marketing expertise; and John Gavin of West Egg Design for creating a welcoming website for readers to land on. A special hug of thanks to Julie Burford, my dear friend, neighbor, and cooking buddy for being there with a nourishing bowl of soup, culinary input, and a willing ear; my friend Bridget Sekera, for her unyielding support during tough times and valuable feedback on the revised recipes; and Jill Leiner, for her lifelong friendship and willingness to make a pot of Magic Mineral Broth at a moment's notice.

All the chocolate chunk cookies in the land could not begin to cover the amount of gratitude I owe to Mat Edelson, an unbelievably gifted writer and storyteller who has been artfully pulling thoughts out of my head for more than a dozen years now.

I know your mother would have been proud of your incredible contributions to both editions of this book.

Thanks to the following people for their never-ending support of my work: Waz Thomas, for his friendship, and picking up the phone to make a call that would change the rest of my life; Michael Lerner, founder of Commonweal's Cancer Help program, for guidance and support; Claire Hart, a fabulous cook and culinary alchemist; Lenore Lefer, my culinary muse, who continues to give me more than a cup of her sage wisdom and support; Michael Broffman and the Pine Street Clinic family, with special thanks to the ever-supportive Louise; everyone at the Center for Mind Body Medicine, and the faculty of Food As Medicine, with a special thanks to James Gordon, MD, Kathie Swift, MS, RD, LDN, and Susan Lord, MD, for bringing the art and science of food and nourishment to an ever-growing audience. And thanks to the effervescent Jo Cooper for her passion and enthusiasm, which nourishes everyone.

I'm also grateful to Barbara and Jay Katz, my parents, for their love and encouragement throughout my journey; my brother Jeff Katz, my nephew and niece Harry and Amelia; to Bella, my very discerning kitchen dog; and to my husband Gregg Kellogg, whose presence in my life has made each day richer and more meaningful.

And, finally, thank you to the clients, students, and readers who have allowed me into their kitchens, pantries, and hearts.

Introduction

I'm betting you could use a little joy in your life right about now. I know one such blissful bundle. It's called the power of "yum," that moment of convergence where smell, taste, and mind align to create an involuntary spasm of vocal delight.

PUTTING YUM TO WORK FOR YOU OR A LOVED ONE IS WHAT THIS BOOK IS ALL ABOUT. Your doctor may be too concerned with your "serious" health issues to spend much time fretting about your taste buds. That's a shame, because those blessed buds are often knocked for a loop by both cancer and its treatments. When those buds get roughed up, there goes your sense of yum.

It doesn't have to be that way. This book is about reconnecting with an old, trusted pal who cheered you up, allowed you to share laughter and love with your family, and turned total strangers into friends. I'm talking, of course, about an outrageously delicious, nutritious plate of food.

You know that there's magic in preparing and sharing a magnificent meal. And at a moment in life when nothing may feel in your control, taking the time to create a simple, delicious dish can be a lifeline, a reaffirmation of your humanity.

What follows are all the tools you need to replace ennui with inspiration and get your creative culinary juices flowing again. The meals you create will have a power that goes beyond mere measurements on a nutritional chart. You'll find that these meals, created to be enjoyed by all who sit around your table, build community and nurture those who keep your spirits aloft: friends, spouse, lover, neighbors, children. This book is for them as well, a place they can turn to with confidence.

It can be daunting cooking for someone with cancer. A favorite meal suddenly is approached by caregivers with the kind of trepidation normally reserved for crossing a minefield. "She loves walnuts with her salad, but the doctor said no nuts." "He goes wild for my fudge brownies, but I've heard sugar can feed cancer." "She's suddenly so finicky." "I can't believe that the smell of tuna fish now makes him nauseous." It's enough to make caregivers throw up their hands in despair and frustration. How do I know? Because on a personal and professional level, I've "been there, done that."

Several years ago, before I embarked on the culinary odyssey that led to this book, my father was diagnosed with throat cancer. The radiation treatments made swallowing nearly impossible. Now there's only one thing you need to know about my dad. He loves food. He lives food. In fact, he made his living in the food business. And there he stood, tears in his eyes, wondering how he'd ever be able to enjoy another meal: "Bec, what am I going to do?" moaned Dad. "Food is the platform of my life!"

I felt utterly helpless. Forget that I was a professionally trained chef running one of Northern California's premiere organic restaurants. What did I know about feeding someone with cancer? I did the best I could—cold fruit smoothies became a staple for him—but there was no one place I could go to find soups, salads, entrées, desserts, snacks, and quick pick-me-ups that were, for lack of a better term, cancer-compatible. That's why these recipes are unique. Every recipe is built around ingredients that taste fantastic (that's the hook!); bolster the immune system; are easy to digest; and work well with numerous healthy substitutions.

These recipes weren't developed overnight. Actually, they wouldn't have been developed at all if I had obeyed the "rules" for feeding cancer patients. I remember bringing my very first client, Shannon, what I thought a cancer patient should eat. My choices were based upon the limited medical literature on the subject. I showed up with bland puréed carrot soup and boring miso soup. I knew these offerings were a palatable snooze-fest, but I figured I'd better behave. Shannon thought otherwise. "You know," she said the next time she saw me, "I'm really craving something a little more . . ."— she searched for the right word that wouldn't hurt my feelings—"uh, exciting."

To my ears that was like getting a papal blessing. I raced out Shannon's door and headed straight for the farmers' market. There I grabbed every fresh and seasonable vegetable I could find. Within an hour I was back in Shannon's kitchen. A few minutes later everything I bought went into the pot along with a layer of spices. In a blink the pot began boiling and heavenly smells wafted through the house. In glided Shannon, following her nose. "That," she said, inhaling deeply over the pot, "is more like it."

I'm glad to say her response is not unique. I'm blessed to be a visiting chef at Commonweal, one of the nation's most respected cancer wellness programs. At Commonweal I often see patients who've been put on restricted diets by doctors or given a list of what they can and can't eat by a nutritionist. Only one thing is missing: no one has shown them how to creatively translate these ingredients into scrumptious dishes. The result? Many of them stop eating, the last thing they can afford to do when they're sick. Fortunately, I've seen these very same people go absolutely gaga when served meals made from the recipes in this book. One man was astounded as he watched his wife with pancreatic cancer go back for a second helping of carrot ginger soup with cashew cream. "She hasn't eaten this much in weeks!" he whispered to me in wonder.

Just as heartwarming is the clear evidence that these foods inspire a sense of wellness that patients want to re-create again and again. I knew this was true by the fourth day of my first Commonweal retreat. One by one, curious patients started showing up in my kitchen. I put them to work peeling, washing, and playing. Their fear of the kitchen quickly melted away, replaced with delight. As I watched my three new helpers make nori rolls, I imagined a doctor suddenly sticking his head in my kitchen and saying something like, "Don't you know these people are sick?" To which I would reply to the doctor, "Tell that to them."

It is this connection to wellness through food that is the subtext here, the same connection that can grow and encompass community as people hopefully move from sickness back to health. One of the most gratifying aspects of writing this book has been hearing from cancer support groups. Many use *One Bite at a Time* as a focal point for coming together, trying the recipes and bringing them to others who could benefit from both the food and the love. At one end of the spectrum is someone like Shannon, who used these recipes to reach out to caregivers when she was feeling zapped from treatment. "Everybody wants to help, but they don't know how. They want to bring you food. They realize that's something they can do, but the trouble is they'll bring anything or what they're having for dinner," says Shannon. "If you can say 'Here are the recipes I like, if you want to try to do something like this,' that helps. Because I wouldn't have made it if my family and friends hadn't taken care of me."

On the other end is Jen, a breast cancer survivor and food writer who loves to cook. Jen is always looking for tasty dishes that will nourish herself and her family. She knew she was on the right track when she whipped up my Taxicab Yellow Tomato Soup for her husband, Ty. Jen could've spouted nutritional facts about the soup until she was blue in the face and Ty would've just yawned. It was the taste that blew him away. "It's been dubbed the moaner soup, because when you taste it, it does make you moan," laughs Jen. She recalls that Ty took one sip and swooned. "He went 'ummmmmm. I had forgotten how much I like tomato soup. Ahhhh!'"

Taste is what it's really all about. I love the way one of my colleagues, Michael Broffman, puts it: "Any food that doesn't taste good can't be good for you." Michael is right in one sense. It's hard to stick with any cuisine that doesn't hug your taste buds, regardless of its health benefits. But I'd go a step further: Everything about the process of eating can be fun, from going to a farmers' market to turning your kitchen into a haven for your culinary creativity to serving your meals in beautiful bowls. Of course, what brings it all together is the payoff: wrapping your mouth around a meal and feeling that shudder of ecstasy rushing through your body.

I'll let you in on another secret. This isn't a diet book. The word diet makes me break out in a cold sweat. It always seems like you're giving up way more than you get from a diet. Who needs that?

In this book you'll find vegetables, fruits, sweets, poultry, and fish. They're all here, presented in sensible ways that take advantage of the nutrition, taste, and immunity-building properties in every morsel of yum.

Some say my cuisine employs a "flexitarian" approach. That's a term I like. To me, a flexitarian is someone who knows how to substitute tasty, healthy foods for items that either common sense or their doctor says they should avoid. Becoming a flexitarian is vital for your physical and mental health. I mean, it's tough enough being sick, but it's downright depressing when your doctor starts telling you, "Spicy foods? I'd prefer you don't. Dairy? I'd pass on that, too." Normally such restrictions are the equivalent of being put in culinary jail with no chance of parole. But that's often not the case when you learn to be a flexitarian.

Once I show you both the wide range of healthy foods at your disposal and how to prepare them,

you'll be amazed at how much your culinary universe will expand. You'll discover substitutes that re-create the taste and texture of those "forbidden" foods. You'll learn to make delicious sweets without refined sugar; satiating creamy soups that are dairy-free and power packed with nutrients; and stews that satisfy carnivorous cravings with just a few ounces of poultry; and, perhaps best of all, you'll get up close and comfortable with your vegetables (the taste will leave you no choice!).

In short, I'm not going to tell you what to eat.

I'd rather show you how to use the best and healthiest organic ingredients that protect your body while providing an explosion of flavor. That's right, I said 'organic.' Now don't freak out. If you don't want to use organics, you don't have to. All of the recipes in this book can be made and thoroughly enjoyed with conventionally grown fruits, vegetables, and meats available in any supermarket. But organics have become so popular over the last few years that you're likely to find them in your favorite grocery store, affordably priced, and often placed side-by-side with their conventionally grown cousins.

I can quote you chapter and verse about why organic foods are better for you than nonorganic foods—more cancer-fighting nutrients, less exposure to nasty pesticides, and so on—but here's the only thing you really need to know: organics taste better. They're fresher. And, if you shop at a farmers' market, they're often grown right in your community. Think of it this way: I'm a chef, and I want my food to taste the best it possibly can. And if your taste buds have been desensitized by cancer treatments, you need that extra burst of flavor in every dish. That's why I use organics whenever possible. Often this little fact blows my clients away, as they realize that healthy eating also tastes wonderful. In short, the days of healthy food resembling bland hippie gruel are gone. So many varieties of organics are now available that they dovetail wonderfully with a flexitarian approach covering many cuisines. "I don't feel deprived, I don't feel like I'm bored, I don't feel like I'm on a narrow path at all," says another of my clients, Andrea. She's a cancer survivor who subsisted on ice cream and yams before she learned how to cook.

"I didn't know how to nourish myself before," says Andrea, who adopted a flexitarian approach that let her flex her culinary muscles. She started with these concepts and is now translating them into her own recipes. "This," says Andrea, "is the first time I feel I can nourish myself and other people."

And I say, "Isn't that what it's all about?"

How to Use This Book

Let's get down to a little learning and help you get the most out of this book. All you need is your taste buds to participate. Even if your buds aren't working perfectly, we'll show you how to get your buds and appetite back.

I've always felt that the more people understand about food from seed to table, the more they enjoy learning to cook. You may want to jump right to the recipes, and that's fine. I've tried to take out as much of the intimidating foodie language as possible. Those things I couldn't take out I explain in a section called Culinary Terms of Endearment.

Personally, I hope you'll be motivated to delve a little deeper into the book. I'd like to be your culinary tour guide on what I promise will be a delightful adventure. I've put together chapters and sidebars that cover everything I teach to my clients and students in cooking classes and home sessions. These include:

• How Friends and Family Can Help. This chapter is vital for caregivers who cook for people who are sick.

• Sustainable Nourishment. Learn a delicious way of eating and living that builds the immune system.

• Nutrition at a Glance. If you want to know about all those fun phytochemicals, minerals, and vitamins in each recipe, this is the place to turn.

• Reinventing and reorganizing your pantry in Pantry Rehabilitation. Get out those garbage bags. This can be like dumpster diving.

• Resource Guide. This information will help you find organic produce and poultry as well as other products we love.

• The Big O. These sidebar points provide information about specific organic ingredients and their health benefits.

• Shopping the farmers' markets in season. It's fun, it's informative, and it's colorful. Plus, there's something to be said for looking in the eye of the person who grows your food.

• Nutritional analyses. I break down each recipe's calories and nutritional components to give you an awareness of what's in each well-balanced dish.

I've placed all the chapters after the recipes, with one very important exception. Following this introduction, you'll find a chapter called The FASS Factor: Tricks for Getting to Yum!

If there's only one chapter you read in this book, it should be this one. Using simple language, this chapter will teach you everything I know about making any meal taste delicious. I'll put it this way: As far as I'm concerned, I need to know addition to do math, the alphabet to write, and FASS to cook.

I promise that FASS will help you balance the taste of any dish you're making. As you go through the recipes, you'll see references to FASS and how it applies. To me, looking at the recipes without first reading about FASS is like going to the opera and passing on the libretto. The more you know, the more you can get out of the experience.

As for the recipes, this really is a community cookbook. Everything you see here has been tried—and often developed—in partnership with my friends and clients. Their insights and experiences over the past four years have shown me what works and what doesn't. There's a refreshing honesty in most of the kitchens I visit, which is reflected in many of the headnotes and sidebars that accompany the recipes. People are up-front about their fears, foibles, and frustrations surrounding food. This is especially true of people who know they have to eat, who want to eat, but can't figure out how to reconnect with food. These dishes serve as a bridge to that place where illness is displaced by the sheer exhilaration of taste. Getting there is partly my job, partly yours. I can show you the way, but I assure you the power of food to heal leaps exponentially when you're the one preparing it.

To that end, think of me not as a cook, but rather as a culinary translator, helping you build a bridge from the gray world of illness and medicine to the technicolor universe of delicious, nutritious meals . . . one bite at a time.

Culinary Assumptions

- Cooking with Oil: Heat the pan first, then add your oil. That way the oil will heat up quicker with less danger of overheating, smoking up the house, and creating free-radicals, those pesky critters that can damage the immune system.

- Spice Combining: If you don't have a certain spice that's called for in your spice cabinet, fret not. The dish will turn out fine. Common spices used in this book are allspice, cumin, cinnamon, and ginger.

- Salt: When I call for salt, I am referring to sea salt with its 80 plus minerals. Sea salt is much tastier than table salt, which has been bleached and has a bitter aftertaste.

- Olive Oil: I am referring to extra virgin olive oil.

- Gluten Intolerance: Non-gluten products can easily be substituted in recipes calling for gluten. Check out the updated Resource Guide for more information.

- Lactose Intolerance: In recipes that call for a lactose product, you can substitute unsweetened soy or rice milk for milk, and coconut or olive oil for butter.

- Tamari: In recipes using tamari (a wheat-free soy sauce), I am calling for low sodium tamari. It's easily found next to the full throttle bottle.

- Organics: Use organic ingredients whenever possible, especially when it comes to animal protein, such as chicken, eggs, and dairy, as well as particular fruits and vegetables. I've highlighted the times when using organic ingredients is particularly important (look for sidebars marked "The Big O").

- I also recommend you use earth-friendly cleaning products in your home, especially dishwashing detergent and liquid.

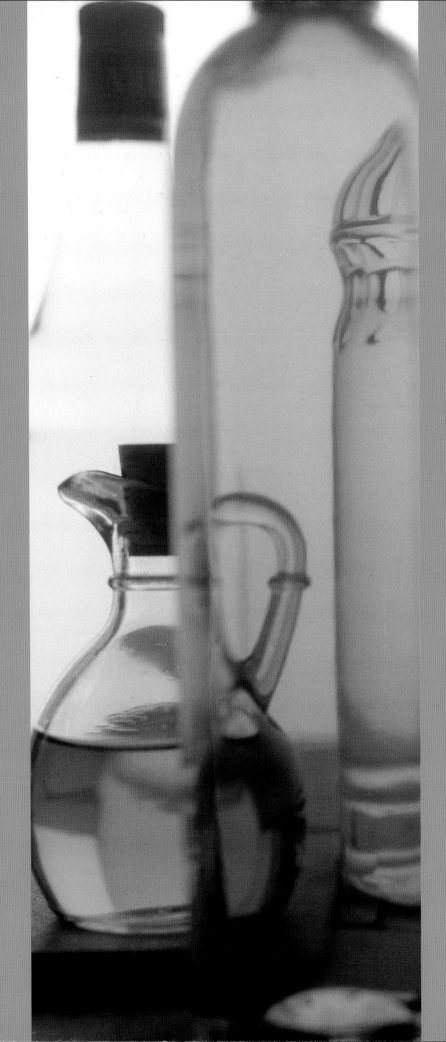

There's a myth — widely perpetuated by chefs — that the ability to differentiate tastes and thus make food taste great is a gift the gods have bestowed on but a few lucky souls.

To which I say, "not true!"

I THINK WE ALL HAVE AN INNATE, ACCURATE SENSE OF TASTE. Chances are your ancestors prospered because they could taste the difference between edible and poisonous berries and between fresh and rotten meat and vegetables. It seems to me you're asking to get tossed out of the gene pool permanently if you're trying to flee from a saber-toothed tiger while suffering from food poisoning.

Given this anthropological evidence, I'm amazed at how little faith people have in their ability to judge flavors. In my experience, cooks new to the kitchen always hem and haw when I ask them how a food tastes and what can be added to improve a dish. And if that cook is someone who is battling cancer, when I ask them to taste a dish in progress they'll almost always say, "I can't taste right."

On the surface there's some truth in that assertion. Cancer treatments — chemo, radiation, and some medications — can sometimes deaden taste buds. Still, I've yet to meet a single person — ill or otherwise — who couldn't be taught how to trust their taste buds. Once that lightbulb goes on, they discover they possess the ability to turn a mediocre dish into a fabulous one. All they needed were the tools and a little education on how to use the tool kit. That's what I gave them. That's what I want to give you.

The magic acronym for learning how to trust your taste buds is FASS; it stands for fat, acid, salt, and sweet. One of my clients, Gary Bang, came up with the acronym when I was going on and on about how the trick to getting any dish to taste right is to balance out its fat, acid, salt, and sweet content. And while I'd like to take credit for FASS, there's really nothing new about the idea of balancing tastes. It's what experienced cooks do, giving it as little conscious thought as a great pianist gives to her breathing when she's performing Schubert to a sold-out house.

I can send you into the kitchen with only four ingredients that will balance any dish and make its natural flavors soar. They are:

- Extra virgin olive oil (your fat)
- Lemon juice (your acid)
- Sea salt (your salt)
- Grade B organic maple syrup (your sweet)

Learn to use these four ingredients and you'll make that once-insurmountable leap from "Hmmm, this needs a little something" to "That's it; *it's perfect!*"

To put FASS to work for you, never forget the number one rule: You must give yourself permission to become a tasting fool. At every step, *every* time you add an ingredient or cook it to release its flavor, you must taste, taste, taste. It's the only proper way to correct a dish's course. Waiting until the end to taste and make changes is like closing the barn door after the horse has already bolted; it's not going to work. Besides, we culinary alchemists love witnessing our ingredients being transformed by the heat into heady creations.

Meet the Band

Now let's introduce the members of the ensemble and explain a bit about the effects they have on your taste buds.

FAT

Fats take food on a magic carpet ride across your palate. That's important because your tongue contains different islands of taste buds. Sweet taste buds tend to gather at the tip of the tongue, while bitter buds congregate toward the back of the mouth. The coating action of fat allows flavors to spread around the tongue and mouth so that they can be fully tasted. Fat also adds some heft to a dish, and its presence leaves us feeling satiated. That's why a little fat goes a long way. Cold-pressed extra virgin olive oil is always my fat of choice because of its nice, clean taste.

ACID

Acids break down the tissues and fibers in vegetables and meats, allowing all those savory juices to run wild. Acids—especially citric acids, which are the acids I'm referring to in FASS—are sour, and they act as an excellent counterbalance to sweet flavors in a dish. Lemons and limes are my acids of choice, but many vinegars, including brown rice, red wine, and balsamic, also fill the bill quite nicely.

SALT

I love the way my friend Gary Bang summarizes a common misconception about salt. "You put salt on your eggs and they taste salty and that's what salt is for." No, no, no, no, no! When used in cooking, real salt—that is, sea salt—is used not to impart its own taste, but rather to unlock the flavor of every food it comes in contact with. As with acids, sea salt crystals act like tiny scrubbing bubbles that release flavors. There is no substitute for sea salt. Basic table salt won't do. It's been bleached of all its elements (save added iodine) and has a slightly

bitter taste. Sea salt is a healthier salt, with more than eighty minerals and elements from the sea. Two last notes on salt for the scientifically inclined: The latest studies suggest that sodium does not cause hypertension, although it may somewhat increase blood pressure. My sense is that informed physicians are leaning toward a "moderation is okay" approach. Another piece of sea salt research may especially interest people with compromised or weakened taste buds. It suggests that sodium stimulates and improves the conductivity of electrical current in nerve cells. Talk about putting a charge in your taste buds!

SWEET

Sweet is the siren song of food. Tease these taste buds, which stand front and center on your tongue, and the brain screams "more, more, more!" This is a vital sensory response for people with cancer. They're not likely to take more than one bite of any dish to which they don't have an immediate positive response. That's not to say you should load up on the sweet, because that's not the goal. Balance is. That's why I use only Grade B organic maple syrup. It's incredibly flavorful, far healthier than refined sugar, and does a marvelous job cutting the acid and bitterness in any dish. Honey, brown rice syrup, and agave nectar all also work in a pinch.

Ready to play with your food? Good. Honing your buds requires a lot of trial and error in the kitchen. I know you don't believe it now, but eventually you'll get so good at FASS that you'll throw a dish's taste off on purpose just to see if you can rebalance it. You'll lusciously succeed . . . and once your friends find this out, they'll call you every time they mess up a recipe.

When I teach people how to use FASS, I often use a soup built from scratch. Why? Because we're taking a flavorless element—water—and turning it into a bowl of yum. Water's complete lack of any taste makes it much easier for those new to FASS to isolate the flavor of every ingredient they add to the pot. Actually, I'm not initially interested in making students correctly guess what part of FASS needs to be added to make a stock taste right. That's too much pressure to put on them. I'd rather engage and excite them about the cooking process and how it slowly releases taste.

I'll use Magic Mineral Broth as an example. I fill the pot with a hodgepodge of vegetables, set it to simmering, and have people taste the stock every ten to fifteen minutes or so. After their third or fourth taste, I see heads start to bob up and down. That once tasteless water is now beginning to metamorphose. Flavors are being released as well as smells, all of which combine to create an aromatic brew. The color of the stock begins to deepen, a visual sign of catalytic change. Old misperceptions break down under the weight of this sensory evidence; new possibilities emerge. That finished pot of stock no longer looks so impossible to create. I catch people staring at it with a newfound confidence.

Once I see that spark, I know my students are ripe for a little FASS learning. I ask a few questions about the pot of stock we've just made. The dialogue usually goes something like this:

Me: "How does it taste?"

Them: "Okay. Pretty good."

Me: "Okay? Do you want to eat just okay food? Let's make it great. What do you think it needs?"

Them: "Hmmm . . . It needs a little salt."

This is a universal response. Everyone reaches for salt first when something doesn't taste quite right. I fill up a quarter teaspoon with sea salt. My students glance at the spoon, then at the twelve-quart stockpot, and immediately get a skeptical look. I know what they're thinking: "That's not enough salt to make it taste salty."

That's true, but it is enough salt to alter the taste. The salt goes in and they taste the stock again. Now their heads begin nodding in unison.

"Better?" I ask.

"Better!" they agree. The salt is doing its job, releasing the stock's flavor. Many times people want to stop right there, but I want to get them to *yum*! So I ask again, "Does it need something else?"

Usually we'll add a pinch or two more of salt and taste the broth again to determine how much the salt can accomplish without creating a salty taste. Everyone agrees the stock tastes great, but now the game's afoot. Tuned into their taste buds, the students sense something is still missing. They just don't know what that something is.

I do. I reach for a lemon. Remember how I said the acids from a little lemon can make flavor notes ring?

"How about this?" I ask, holding up the lemon. There are more surprised looks. People are thinking of how sour a lemon tastes instead of focusing on its ability to enhance existing flavors. They don't want a sour taste in their stock—and I can't blame them—but they're willing to go along with me. Spritz. Taste. Lip smacks. Even a few gasps of delight.

"Wow. That's it!"

"That is soooo great."

And it is great, as a base. Delicious stock is the foundation for great soup. Still, although this stock is tasty and nutritious, it doesn't have the satiating quality of a meal. Why? Again, remember what FASS stands for. The stock has acid, salt, and some sweet from the juice of the vegetables. What's missing? That's right: fat. Most people make soup using fat-free vegetable stock. This means that the rest of the soup ingredients need to contain some fat to round out the dish.

Here's how the rest of the lesson plays out. For many classes I choose to make Caramelized Sweet Red Onion Soup with the Magic Mineral Broth as stock. I use this combination because it's relatively simple, extremely tasty, and helps me demonstrate FASS in action. In a saucepan we pour some extra virgin olive oil. That's the fat. Then we add onions and a pinch of salt. Again, the salt can't be tasted, but it breaks down the onion, releasing more of its juice. After the onions are golden brown we pour a cup of stock over the onions, reduce the contents to seal in the flavor, and then pour in the rest of the stock. Invariably, someone asks the question I've been waiting for: "I see how we added fat, but where did we add sweetness?"

I put a spoon in their hand and point them to the pot.

"I can't believe onion soup could taste so sweet!" is the inevitable response. I've tricked them a bit by keeping them away from the onions while they cooked, but only to make the point that many vegetables, when allowed to cook properly, produce a luscious, sweet juice.

So now we're almost there. Once again, we go over what's in the soup from a FASS viewpoint. We have our fat, the olive oil. We've added sea salt along the way to our onions. Those onions, in turn, released sweet juice.

"What's missing?"

Everyone points to the lemon. We need a little acid. Just a little more brightness to bring it home. Spritz.

Taste. Incomplete sentences. "Oh! Wow!" Someone's taste buds have just received a serious wake-up call! We have reached yum!

Throughout this book you'll see references to FASS. These include tips on how to balance FASS in stews, salads, and even snacks. It's not a test; I promise you the recipes will taste delicious even if you'd rather not think about FASS. But I hope you do make the effort to think about FASS for a couple of reasons. I look at these recipes as launching points for your own creativity. FASS is a great tool to have at your disposal when you decide it's time to take off on your own culinary wanderings, a kind of global positioning system for your taste buds.

Think about what FASS does and how it pertains to cooking for people with cancer. Let's say their taste buds have been somewhat compromised and they taste only half of what you and I taste. Without attention to FASS, a given meal may have only 75 percent of its potential taste. To you and me that's mediocre but tolerable. But to someone with compromised taste buds that same meal is nearly flavorless, a complete turnoff. After one bite they're done. By optimizing a dish's taste with FASS, that same person is drawn to the food. The bottom line is they eat more. They're nourished. They feel better. For a precious moment, you've helped them reconnect to food, and in turn to life, health, and wellness.

Nothing makes a person feel better, feel more nourished, than a bowl of soup. The very act of making soup—turning plain old water into an enchanting elixir—is culinary alchemy at its finest. Making soup is, literally, a heady experience; as it simmers, steam rises, intoxicatingly engaging the sense of smell, and where the nose goes, the mouth, heart, and tummy are sure to follow.

SOUP IS ALSO INCREDIBLY VERSATILE. Not too hungry? Check out the Magic Mineral Broth. This is the ideal light, nutrient-packed broth for many cancer patients whose appetites have been dragged down by treatment. Looking for something obscenely sumptuous? Head toward the creamy cashmere collection. These dairy-free soups have that luscious slide-right-down-your-throat texture that one associates with milk-based soups (you'll have to look at the recipes to see how we pull it off).

Soups are also wonderful for people who are having trouble digesting whole foods. The cooking process breaks down the crunchy nature of many vegetables, releasing nutrients into the broth. Not up to munching greens? No problem. Throw them in a soup and let the water and the blender do the work for you.

Let's bust a myth about soups here: Contrary to popular belief, they shouldn't be served just off the boil. It's not a matter of heat as much as taste. It's easier to taste a soup when it's warm than when it's boiling hot. Intense heat overwhelms taste buds; instead of reacting to taste, they're recoiling from the temperature. This is true for everyone, but it's especially true for people whose taste has been affected by treatment. Broths can be served at a higher temperature than thicker soups, but I'd let even broths cool a bit before eating them.

Soups also store extremely well. Properly stored in individual airtight containers, soup can last for months in the freezer. That's one long hug.

All-Purpose Chicken Stock

There are two ways to look at chicken stock. From a culinary perspective, it's the base for numerous fine soups and sauces. That's all well and good, and no doubt will earn you an A on your cooking final. Still, I prefer Grandma's take on chicken stock: It's healing. Really. One scientific study showed that chicken soup moved certain colds along faster than mere hot water. Anyone I have ever fed chicken soup to feels nourished. When nothing else will do, fill up a mug with steaming chicken stock and sip. My grandmother called it Jewish penicillin. I call it liquid gold.

6 pounds organic chicken backs, necks, or bones

2 unpeeled medium white onions, coarsely chopped

4 unpeeled carrots, cut into thirds

2 celery stalks, chopped into thirds

6 fresh thyme sprigs

1 large bunch fresh flat-leaf parsley

1 bay leaf

8 black peppercorns

1 teaspoon sea salt

INNER COOK NOTES
Ready to strain the soup? Now visualize this . . . water weighs 8 pounds a gallon and you have a stockpot full of it! Call for help; this may be a two-person job.

Stock can be frozen for up to 3 months. Store stock in various sizes of containers so that you can pull out a small one for deglazing or a larger one to make a pot of soup.

In a stockpot, combine the chicken, onions, carrots, celery, thyme, parsley, bay leaf, peppercorns, and salt. Fill the pot with water to 2 inches below the rim of the pot. Cover and heat over medium-high heat until the water comes to a boil.

Uncover and skim off the scum and the fat that has risen to the surface. Lower the heat so the bubbles just break the surface of the liquid and simmer until the stock tastes rich, about 2 to 3 hours. Get your spoon out; you may want to add a couple generous pinches of salt—one at a time—to taste.

Strain the stock through a fine-mesh sieve or colander lined with unbleached cheesecloth into a clean pot or heat-resistant bowl. Bring to room temperature before covering and storing in the refrigerator. The next day, spoon off and discard any fat that has risen to the surface.

Makes 6 quarts

PER SERVING (1 cup per serving) Calories: 41; Total Fat: 0 g (0 g saturated, 0 g monounsaturated); Carbohydrates: 1 g; Protein: 7 g; Fiber: 0 g; Sodium: 71 mg

Here's a lesson that's better to learn from someone else's experience. A friend made this stock and let it simmer for hours. Heavenly aromas filled her home. With taste buds salivating, she was ready to strain and taste. She brought the pot over to her deep sink and, with a strainer in place, in went the stock. Only problem was, my friend had forgotten to place a pot *underneath* the strainer. Before she could recover, most of the stock had gone right down the drain. The good news? There was enough stock left to give her dogs gravy on their dinner.

Caramelized Sweet Red Onion Soup with Parmesan Crostini

INNER COOK NOTES

If a large sauté pan isn't part of your collection yet, use your stockpot or soup pot. The important thing is to use a wide-bottom pan so the onions cook in a single layer rather than a heap. If you add wine, the alcohol will evaporate during cooking, leaving only the flavor behind. A great salad to complement this soup is the Mixed Greens with Roasted Beets and Avocado Tossed with Orange-Shallot Vinaigrette (page 42).

This may come as a shock, but onions weren't meant to be stinky! The way we take onions from "phew" to "whoaaaa!!!" is by caramelizing them. No, that doesn't mean you coat the onion in caramel. Rather, you use a little heat to prod the onion into giving up its sweet juices. Caramelizing is a technique I love to teach because it's useful in so many recipes. Master the art and your reward will be a fragrant dish the equal of anything you'll eat in a French bistro. Who knew onions could taste so good?

SOUP

2 tablespoons extra virgin olive oil

6 large red onions, halved and sliced $1/2$ inch thick

Pinch of sea salt

2 teaspoons chopped fresh thyme, or 1 teaspoon dried thyme

1 cup red wine (optional)

8 cups Magic Mineral Broth (page 13) or prepared vegetable stock

Pinch of freshly grated nutmeg

PARMESAN CROSTINI

1 sourdough baguette

2 teaspoons extra virgin olive oil

$1/4$ cup freshly grated organic Parmesan cheese (optional)

2 tablespoons finely chopped fresh flat-leaf parsley, for garnish

Preheat the oven to 350°F.

In a large, straight-sided sauté pan, heat the 2 tablespoons of olive oil over medium heat. Add the onions and salt and stir. Decrease the heat to medium-low. Allow the onions to caramelize, about 25 minutes (see Culinary Terms of Endearment, page 150).

When the onions have turned a deep golden brown, stir in the thyme and deglaze with the wine or 1 cup of the broth. The liquid will reduce and intensify in flavor. Add 8 cups of broth and the nutmeg and simmer for 15 minutes.

While the soup is simmering, slice the baguette into $1/4$-inch rounds and place on a baking sheet. Brush the top of each slice lightly with olive oil and sprinkle with cheese. Bake until lightly toasted and the cheese has melted.

Serve the soup in bowls with a crostini floating on top and garnish with the parsley.

Serves 6

PER SERVING Calories: 269; Total Fat: 7 g (0 g saturated, 4 g monounsaturated); Carbohydrates: 46 g; Protein: 7 g; Fiber: 6 g; Sodium: 527 mg

Sometimes it takes some course adjustment to rescue a soup. I was teaching a group of caregivers this recipe when we accidentally added several very large onion peels to the pot. A participant, Monica, recalled what happened: "When we tasted it, well, 'swill' is putting it nicely. The rest of the class was spent learning how to correct the mistake." We diluted the stock by half and added some lemon juice and a tablespoon of Grade B organic maple syrup. Monica adds, "In the end, after much tasting and laughing, we witnessed the magic of turning a pot of bitter stock into a sweet, savory bowl of soup!"

Chicken Soup with Bowtie Pasta

If my chicken stock is Jewish penicillin, this is where Brooklyn meets Bologna. Adding sage and thyme to the mix of chicken and veggies gives this soup an aromatic boost. This simple yet filling soup is ideal for serving in small or large amounts, depending upon one's appetite.

INNER COOK NOTES
If the pasta is al dente before the vegetables are ready, rinse the pasta with cool water to stop the cooking until the vegetables call you and say they're ready to tie it on!

2 tablespoons extra virgin olive oil

1 cup diced yellow onion

$1/4$ teaspoon sea salt

1 cup peeled and diced carrot

1 cup peeled and diced celery

$1/4$ teaspoon dried thyme

$1/4$ teaspoon dried sage

8 cups No-Fuss Roasted Chicken Stock (page 53), All-Purpose Chicken Stock (page 9), or prepared chicken stock

$1/2$ cup shredded or cubed roasted, grilled, or poached organic chicken

1 cup cooked bowtie or other pasta

In a sauté pan, heat the olive oil over medium heat. Add the onions and a pinch of salt and sauté until golden. Add the carrots and celery to the onions with another pinch of salt and sauté for 3 minutes. Add the thyme and sage, stirring to coat the vegetables. Deglaze the pan with $1/2$ cup of the stock. Add the remaining stock and chicken and cook until the vegetables are tender, about 10 minutes.

While the vegetables are simmering, bring a large pot of water to a boil. Add $1/4$ teaspoon salt to the boiling water, add the pasta, and cook until al dente. Drain the pasta and add it to the soup and heat through. Ladle into bowls and serve.

Serves 6

PER SERVING Calories: 621; Total Fat: 33 g (8 g saturated, 14 g monounsaturated); Carbohydrates: 21 g; Protein: 56 g; Fiber: 4 g; Sodium: 369 mg

Chickpea Soup with Caramelized Fennel and Orange Zest

INNER COOK NOTES
For a smooth, creamy soup, put a third of the broth in a blender first, then add the chickpeas. Purée until smooth, serve, and garnish.

I'm thankful that my three Mediterranean cousins, hummus, babaganoush, and falafel brought chickpeas into the culinary mainstream, but most people—unless they've been to Sicily—haven't yet experienced chickpeas floating in a delicate broth. Be sure the fennel and onions turn a luscious golden color before adding the spices to the broth. The orange zest provides both taste and auditory effect: Whoever tastes this soup won't be able to stop a moan of delight from sneaking past their lips.

When you're cooking for someone who doesn't feel well, often you get only one shot at engaging their appetite. They simply don't have the strength to make it through a mediocre meal. One way to increase someone's desire to eat is to engage all their senses. One of my clients told me what sold her on this soup. "I loved the fragrance of the soup as it was cooking. Also, it was pretty."

If whole fennel is hard to find, use celery instead and add a teaspoon of fennel seeds to the onions. Crack the fennel seeds with a mortar and pestle to release their flavor. If you don't have a mortar and pestle and the local apothecary is closed for the night, put the tiny seeds in a food processor and give them a quick pulse or wrap them in a kitchen towel and whack them with a rolling pin.

1 pound fennel bulbs

3 tablespoons fresh lemon juice

2 tablespoons extra virgin olive oil

2 cups diced yellow onions

Pinches of sea salt

4 cloves garlic, minced

1/2 teaspoon dried oregano

1/8 teaspoon ground cinnamon

2 teaspoons grated orange zest

8 cups Magic Mineral Broth (page 13)

4 cups cooked chickpeas or 2 (15-ounce) cans chickpeas, drained, rinsed, and mixed with a spritz of fresh lemon juice and a pinch of salt

1 teaspoon chopped fresh mint, for garnish

1 teaspoon chopped fresh flat-leaf parsley, for garnish

Trim the stems and fronds from the fennel. Cut the bulbs in half, remove the core, cut into quarters, and slice crosswise into thin diagonal slices. Set aside in a bowl of water with a squeeze of lemon juice.

In an 8-quart pot, heat the olive oil. Add the onions and a pinch of salt and sauté over medium heat for about 5 minutes. Add the fennel and a pinch of salt and continue to sauté until both are golden brown and tender. Stir in the garlic, oregano, cinnamon, and orange zest. Cook for 1 minute more.

Deglaze the pan with 1/4 cup of the broth. Capture all the flavor by loosening all the bits on the bottom. Add the remaining broth and bring to a boil. Decrease the heat and simmer for about 15 minutes. Add the chickpeas and simmer for about 5 minutes more.

Taste the soup. Think FASS. You may want to add a squeeze of lemon juice, a generous pinch of salt, or some additional orange zest. Ladle the soup into bowls and garnish each serving with the mint and parsley.

Serves 6

PER SERVING Calories: 309; Total Fat: 7 g (1 g saturated, 4 g monounsaturated); Carbohydrates: 50 g; Protein: 12 g; Fiber: 14 g; Sodium: 296 mg

Magic Mineral Broth™

If all you get out of this book is the information in the FASS chapter and this recipe, I'd be happy. This broth alone can keep people going, especially when they don't particularly want to eat. It's not just a regular vegetable stock. This pot of yum is high in potassium and numerous trace minerals that are often depleted by cancer therapy. Sipping this nutrient-rich stock is like giving your body an internal spa treatment. Drink it like a tea, or use it as a base for all your favorite soups and rice dishes. Don't be daunted by the ingredient list. Simply chop the ingredients in chunks and throw them in the pot, roots, skins, and all.

6 unpeeled carrots, cut into thirds

2 unpeeled medium yellow onions, cut into chunks

1 leek, both white and green parts, cut into thirds

1 bunch celery, including the heart, cut into thirds

5 unpeeled cloves garlic, halved

¹/₂ bunch fresh flat-leaf parsley

4 medium red potatoes with skins on, quartered

2 Japanese or regular sweet potatoes with skins on, quartered

1 Garnet yam with skin on, quartered

1 (8-inch) strip of kombu

2 bay leaves

12 black peppercorns

4 whole allspice or juniper berries

1 tablespoon sea salt

Rinse all of the vegetables well, including the kombu. In a 12-quart or larger stockpot, combine all the ingredients, except the salt. Fill the pot to 2 inches below the rim with water, cover, and bring to a boil.

Remove the lid, decrease the heat to low, and simmer for a minimum of 2 hours. As the stock simmers, some of the water will evaporate; add more if the vegetables begin to peek out. Simmer until the full richness of the vegetables can be tasted. Add the salt and stir.

Strain the stock using a large coarse-mesh strainer (remember to use a heat-resistant container underneath). Bring to room temperature before refrigerating or freezing.

Makes 6 to 7 quarts

PER SERVING Calories: 29; Total Fat: 0 g (0 g saturated, 0 g monounsaturated); Carbohydrates: 6 g; Protein: 0 g; Fiber: 0 g; Sodium: 166 mg

INNER COOK NOTES

If you don't have time to make this broth from scratch, substitute Pacific or Imagine brand vegetable stock, add an equal quantity of water, a piece of kombu, and one potato. Boil for 20 minutes and strain. Magic Mineral Broth can be frozen for up to 6 months in a variety of airtight containers for every use.

A caregiver I know who never cooked tried this recipe for his mother, who was fighting colon cancer at the time. "After I put all the vegetables in the pot and started them simmering, I had to go out of the house for a half hour to get something for Mom. When I got home and opened the front door, I couldn't believe how amazing the house smelled. What was even more incredible was that I had created these smells. Before I left to go home, mom wrote me a small check to cover the cost. I couldn't understand why she thought she had to pay me for this. Then I looked at the "memo" part on the front of the check. Next to it she wrote these words: "Love Soup."

Miso-Ginger Soup with Udon Noodles

Talk about devotion to a recipe: One caregiver ran eight blocks through the streets of New Orleans while the soup was simmering, all so she could find an Asian restaurant that would give her a half teaspoon of sesame oil. The look on her friend's face when she finally tasted the soup made the madcap sprint worth the effort. I guess that's what chefs really mean when they say to add a dash of something.

Remember when you had a stomachache as a kid? Mom's folk remedy was probably a little cottage cheese or tea and toast. Too bad we all didn't have Japanese grandparents. They knew what some of us have finally learned in the last few years: miso soup works wonders. A little miso in hot water makes a delightful tea, especially on those days when the thought of eating a heavy meal doesn't have you doing cartwheels. In this recipe the ginger and lemon add taste without creating tumult in the tummy. Going the full monty with the udon noodles and vegetables turns this soup into a luscious, nutritious meal in a bowl.

4 ounces udon noodles, broken into thirds

8 cups Magic Mineral Broth (page 13)

1 tablespoon extra virgin olive oil

$1/2$ teaspoon sesame oil

1 small yellow onion, thinly sliced

Pinches of sea salt

2 carrots, peeled and sliced into 1-inch matchsticks

2 tablespoons minced fresh ginger

2 tablespoons mirin

$1/4$ cup white miso

2 to 4 tablespoons fresh lemon juice

1 bunch scallions, green and white parts, sliced diagonally

In a 4-quart pot, bring 2 quarts of water to a boil over high heat. Add a pinch of salt and the udon noodles and cook until al dente. Drain and rinse under cold water. Set the noodles aside.

In the same pot, bring the broth to a boil. Lower the heat to maintain a simmer.

While the stock simmers, heat the olive oil and sesame oil over medium heat in a sauté pan. Add the onions and a pinch of salt, lower the heat, and caramelize until golden brown, about 20 minutes. Add the carrots and ginger and sauté for 3 minutes. Deglaze the pan with the mirin and sauté for 1 minute more.

In a small bowl, combine $1/4$ cup of the hot broth with the miso, stirring with a fork until the miso is dissolved. Add the sautéed vegetables, and dissolved miso mixture to the broth. Cover the pot and remove from the heat. Let sit for 2 to 3 minutes.

Add the cooked udon noodles, lemon juice, and scallions to the broth. Serve in small, colorful soup bowls.

Serves 6

PER SERVING Calories: 200; Total Fat: 4 g (0 g saturated, 2 g monounsaturated); Carbohydrates: 35 g; Protein: 6 g; Fiber: 6 g; Sodium: 621mg

Asparagus Soup with Pistachio Cream

Asparagus is daunting to some folks. They look like little trees and some people dubiously approach cooking them as if they've been asked to sauté a redwood. A wise Italian cook gave me the inside skinny on preparing asparagus. She said it's best to peel away the tough, stringy outer layer to expose the sweet flesh beneath. When they're finished roasting—and we're not talking a lot of time here, maybe fifteen minutes— you'll have a real treat. Roasted asparagus is so naturally sweet it's like eating candy. I know you probably don't believe me now, but try a piece as you take the asparagus out of the oven and you'll be lucky if the stalks make it to the blender for soup.

INNER COOK NOTES
Adding pistachio cream puréed with a tablespoon of fresh mint makes this a yummy, creamy spring soup that can be served warm or chilled.

Substitute zucchini when asparagus is out of season. Roasting brings out zucchini's sweetness.

SOUP

2 pounds asparagus

3 tablespoons extra virgin olive oil

$1/4$ teaspoon sea salt

1 cup diced yellow onion

2 chopped leeks, white part only

1 cup peeled and diced Yellow Finn or Yukon gold potatoes

1 tablespoon diced shallot

2 cloves garlic, chopped

8 cups Magic Mineral Broth (page 13) or prepared vegetable stock

1 recipe Pistachio Cream (page 116)

Freshly grated nutmeg, for garnish

Preheat the oven to 425°F. Snap off the tough ends of the asparagus and place the stalks in a single layer on a large sheet pan. Drizzle the asparagus with 1 tablespoon of the olive oil and the $1/4$ teaspoon salt. Roast for about 10 minutes (less if the asparagus is thin, more if the stalks are thick), shaking the sheet pan to turn the asparagus once during roasting. Reserve the asparagus tips as a garnish.

Heat the remaining 2 tablespoons olive oil in an 8-quart pot over medium heat. Add the onions, leeks, and a pinch of salt. Sauté for 3 minutes, then add the potatoes, shallots, and a pinch of salt. Stir occasionally, allowing the potatoes to soften and the onions to turn golden. Add the garlic and sauté for 30 seconds. When the mixture begins to stick to the bottom of the pot, deglaze with 1 cup of the broth. Continue to cook, reducing the liquid by half. Add 7 more cups of the stock and simmer for 5 minutes.

In batches, purée the soup in a blender, adding the liquid first, then the roasted asparagus stalks. Blend until smooth. Strain through a chinois or a fine-mesh strainer, using the back of a wooden spoon to push the liquid through. This will create that cashmere-like texture. If the soup is too thick, add more broth $1/2$ cup at a time.

Stir the pistachio cream into the soup. Ladle the soup into bowls and garnish with the reserved asparagus tips and freshly grated nutmeg. Serve with Parmesan Crostini (page 10).

Serves 6

PER SERVING Calories: 313; Total Fat: 17 g (2 g saturated, 10 g monounsaturated); Carbohydrates: 32 g; Protein: 10 g; Fiber: 9 g; Sodium: 433 mg

Carrot-Ginger Soup with Cashew Cream

It's easy to slightly alter or intensify a taste for someone whose taste buds have been compromised by cancer treatment. I taught Mary Jane and her husband how to make this soup. Willard tasted it and liked it, but Mary Jane, who was undergoing chemo, couldn't taste much. I whipped out my lemon squeezer and added a touch of lemon juice and salt, two ingredients that immediately brighten a dish. Mary Jane took a sip. Better, but not yet great. That's when I topped the soup with the cashew cream. Mary Jane tasted, and her "yummms" filled the room. After she finished she looked at me and said, "This is my new teddy bear soup."

The Big O: Want to experience a vegetable that taste likes candy? Find organic baby carrots at your local farmers' market. In addition to the usual benefits of going organic— less pesticide exposure, better nutrient profile—the prep work is easier. Just give them a quick rinse and leave the skins on (if you're using conventionally grown carrots, please wash and peel them first).

This versatile soup can be prepared either with Magic Mineral Broth or using the carrot cooking liquid as your stock. The ginger adds an agreeable pep, but the real showstopper is the Cashew Cream. Your taste buds will thank you.

SOUP

2 tablespoons extra virgin olive oil

2 cups chopped yellow onions

3 pounds carrots washed and cut into 1-inch pieces

2 teaspoons grated fresh ginger

$^1/_2$ teaspoon curry powder

$^1/_4$ teaspoon ground cumin

$^1/_8$ teaspoon ground cinnamon

$^1/_8$ teaspoon ground allspice

$^1/_8$ teaspoon ground coriander

1 small pinch of red pepper flakes

8 cups cold water or Magic Mineral Broth (page 13)

1 teaspoon sea salt

$^1/_8$ teaspoon maple syrup (optional)

CASHEW CREAM

1 cup raw cashews

1 cup water

2 teaspoons fresh lemon juice

$^1/_4$ teaspoon sea salt

Pinch of freshly grated nutmeg

In a 6- to 8-quart pot, heat the olive oil over medium heat. Add the onions with a pinch of salt and sauté until golden. Add the carrots, ginger, curry, cumin, cinnamon, allspice, coriander, and red pepper flakes and stir to combine. Deglaze the pan with 1 cup of water or broth, then add the remaining 7 cups of liquid and 1 teaspoon of salt. Cook until the carrots are tender, about 20 minutes.

In a blender, purée the soup in batches, adding the cooking liquid first and then the carrots. Blend until very smooth. Add additional liquid to reach the desired thickness. Return to the pot, add the maple syrup, and reheat slowly. Think FASS and taste. Does it need a squeeze of lemon, a pinch or two of salt, or a drizzle of maple syrup?

To make the cashew cream, grind the cashews in a mini food processor or nut grinder (some blenders are not powerful enough to turn nuts into cream, so we give them a head start). If you have a Vita-Mix (page 153), skip this step. Put the water in a blender. Add the ground cashews, lemon juice, salt, and nutmeg. Blend until very smooth, about 3 minutes. To serve, ladle the soup into bowls and drizzle Cashew Cream on top.

Serves 6

PER SERVING Calories: 207; Total Fat: 11 g (2 g saturated, 6 g monounsaturated); Carbohydrates: 25 g; Protein: 5 g; Fiber: 6 g; Sodium: 491 mg

Emerald City Soup

I first made this soup during a retreat. It started out as luscious broccoli soup, but I didn't have enough broccoli to feed twenty people. I realized this 15 minutes before lunch was to be served, so I looked around the kitchen and spotted green dino kale just begging to be added. I trusted my instincts and was blessed with a cross between culinary alchemy and a nutritionist's dream: two of the most powerful cancer-fighting foods merged in a tasty and easy-to-digest soup. Gotcha! This soup has become my secret weapon. You just had two-plus servings of greens, and that was before you went back for seconds.

$3/_4$ teaspoon sea salt

2 large bunches broccoli, cut into florets and stems peeled and cut into chunks

2 tablespoons extra virgin olive oil

1 cup chopped yellow onion

2 cloves garlic, minced

$1/_8$ teaspoon red pepper flakes

1 bunch kale, stemmed and chopped into small pieces (about 3 cups)

8 cups Magic Mineral Broth (page 13)

$1/_4$ cup fresh lemon juice

$1/_4$ teaspoon maple syrup (optional)

In a large pot, bring 6 cups of water to a boil with $1/_2$ teaspoon of the salt. Place the broccoli in a metal colander and plunge it into the boiling water. Cook just until tender but firm and bright green, 30 seconds. Immediately immerse the broccoli in an ice water bath to retain its bright color.

Heat the olive oil in a medium sauté pan over medium heat. Add the onions and a pinch of salt and sauté for about 10 minutes, just until the onions are translucent and begin to turn golden. Add the garlic and red pepper flakes. Continue sautéing for 30 seconds, until aromatic. Add the kale and a pinch of salt. Cook for 1 minute, until the kale turns bright green. Immediately remove the pan from the heat.

In a blender, add one-third of the broth, one-third of the broccoli, and the kale mixture. Blend until smooth. When the color changes from pale green to vivid emerald, that's your cue to turn off the blender. Pour into a clean pot and repeat until all of the ingredients have been blended. Add the lemon juice, the remaining $1/_4$ teaspoon salt, and the maple syrup to the last blender batch. Stir and reheat the soup very slowly over low heat. Serve immediately in colorful soup bowls or soup mugs. If you need to make it in advance, heat it slowly or it will lose its emerald green color and turn muddy.

Serves 6

PER SERVING Calories: 155; Total Fat: 5 g (0 g saturated, 3 g monounsaturated); Carbohydrates: 24 g; Protein: 6 g; Fiber: 7 g; Sodium: 576 mg

INNER COOK NOTES
Emerald City Soup does not freeze well, as it will not retain its vibrant green color. The soup can, however, be kept for 1 to 2 days in the refrigerator.

This is a favorite soup at the clinic where I teach. Many of the clinic's clients are battling breast cancer. This comment came from one of those courageous women. "I never knew what to do with kale. It wasn't even on my culinary radar screen. But I really loved this soup when I tasted it in class. I was so excited by the thought of eating something that not only was good for me but also tasted and looked good that I attempted the soup the next day. I guess I was a little overzealous when I put my ingredients in the blender. I filled the blender, put the lid on, and pressed the button. The top flew off and emerald green splashed all over the counter, the wall, and the ceiling. My husband said it looked like I was having fun in the kitchen making spinning art." The moral? Don't fill the blender more than two-thirds full.

Sweet Potato–Coconut Soup

As treatments during a chemotherapy cycle progress, some people find that their fatigue stretches out for several days at a time. The need for energy without effort peaks. My client Shannon says she found gentle nourishment in this dish during this time. "The first couple of days after chemo, I had the sweet potato soup with ginger. The ginger helped my nausea, and the sweet potatoes and yams were easy for me to digest."

This healing concoction is a double shot, combining the broth from the Poached Coconut Ginger Salmon (page 59) and sweet potato comfort. Many of my clients crave sweet potatoes, which aren't really potatoes at all but rather an edible root from the morning glory family. Enzymes in the root convert starch into sweetness as it grows, yet the root still retains plenty of nutrition, including vitamin B_6 and potassium.

8 cups Magic Mineral Broth (page 13)

2 (14.5-ounce) cans coconut milk

3 (1-inch) pieces fresh ginger

2 shallot bulbs, halved and bruised

3 kaffir lime leaves (page 140) or 1 teaspoon zest of a lime

1 stalk lemongrass, cut in chunks and bruised

$1/4$ teaspoon salt

3 sweet potatoes or yams, peeled and cut into 1-inch cubes

Squeeze of fresh lime juice

Chopped fresh mint, for garnish

Chopped fresh cilantro, for garnish

Shaved coconut, toasted, for garnish

In a 6-quart pot, bring the broth, coconut milk, ginger, shallots, lime leaves, lemongrass, and $1/4$ teaspoon salt to a slow boil over medium heat. Let the ingredients infuse their flavor into the liquid for about 20 minutes. Decrease the heat to low and continue to let the broth develop for another 30 to 40 minutes; it will be worth the wait. Remove the shallots, lime leaves, and lemongrass with a slotted spoon. Add the sweet potatoes and turn the heat back up to medium. Cook the sweet potatoes until tender, about 15 minutes.

In a blender, purée small batches of the broth and potatoes until smooth. Remember not to fill your blender more than two-thirds full and put a towel over the top! Repeat until all the soup is blended. Reheat, ladle into soup bowls, drizzle with the lime juice, and garnish with the mint, cilantro, and some toasted shaved coconut. Yum!

Serves 6

PER SERVING Calories: 370; Total Fat: 29 g (25 g saturated, 1 g monounsaturated); Carbohydrates: 26 g; Protein: 4 g; Fiber: 6 g; Sodium: 276 mg

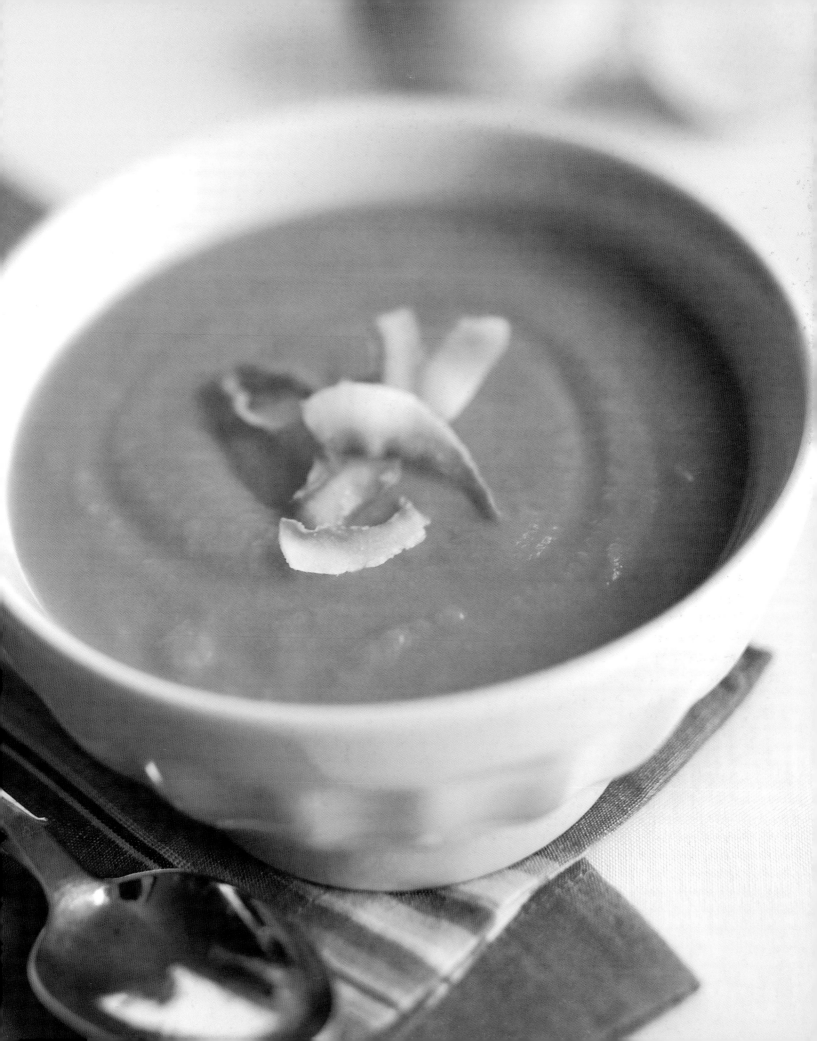

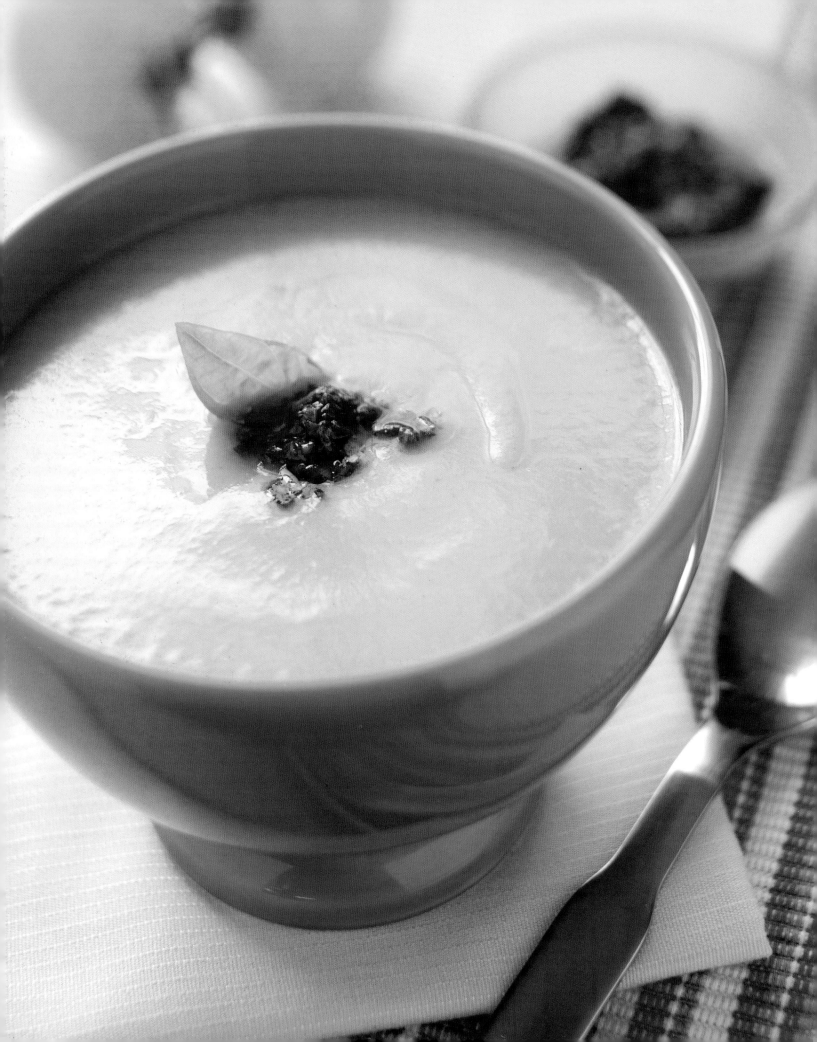

Taxicab Yellow Tomato Soup with Fresh Basil Pesto

That's right: yellow *tomatoes. Never had one? You will now. The little yellow gems are less acidic then their red brethren (although if red is all you have in the house, they'll do). I know this may sound corny, but yellow tomatoes make me feel like I'm eating sunshine. Then again, this* is *a late summertime soup. The roasting process unlocks the tomato's natural sweetness, while the blending makes for a smooth, creamy soup.*

8 pounds yellow heirloom tomatoes, halved

2 tablespoons extra virgin olive oil

1 teaspoon sea salt

1 to 2 cups Magic Mineral Broth (page 13) or prepared vegetable stock (optional), as needed

PESTO

1/4 cup coarsely chopped fresh basil

1 tablespoon extra virgin olive oil

Pinch of sea salt

2 teaspoons cold water

Squeeze of fresh lemon juice

(page 13)

Preheat the oven to 425°F.

Gently squeeze the halved tomatoes in your hand to remove excess seeds. Place the tomatoes in a bowl and toss with the olive oil and salt. Arrange the tomatoes, cut side down, in a single layer on rimmed sheet pans. Roast for 20 to 30 minutes, until the skins are just browning and the juices are bubbling. Remove from the oven, cool, and lift off the skins.

In batches, add the tomatoes with their juice to a blender and purée until smooth. Pour the blended tomatoes through a strainer into a clean pot. Use the back of a wooden spoon to push the liquid through the strainer and discard any remaining skins.

The roasted tomatoes give off so much juice that the purée shouldn't be too thick. If it is, add the broth 1/2 cup at a time to achieve the desired consistency.

To make the pesto, process the basil in a food processor while drizzling in the olive oil. Add a pinch of salt and the water. Taste and add a squeeze of lemon juice.

Reheat the soup slowly over medium-low heat. Serve in a boldly colored soup bowl with a dollop of the pesto. Yum to the eye and the tum! This soup can be eaten at room temperature, chilled, or warmed.

Serves 6

PER SERVING Calories: 156; Total Fat: 9 g (1 g saturated, 5 g monounsaturated); Carbohydrates: 19 g; Protein: 6 g; Fiber: 5 g; Sodium: 584 mg

INNER COOK NOTES
Some tomatoes are juicier than others; you may need to drain the tomato juice into a bowl during the roasting process.

Just about everyone I know who likes tomatoes hates the seeds, and with good reason: tomato seeds, especially in a blended soup, may add a bitter aftertaste.

Cooking shouldn't be serious. Sometimes it can even be hilarious. We were showing people how to make this soup in a class. First we passed out the soup without the pesto. Everyone tried it and nodded politely. Then we added the pesto and they all tasted it again. From the back of the room came a moan from a woman. Actually, it was more than a moan. Kind of like the note of ecstasy Meg Ryan hit in the diner in *When Harry Met Sally*. My male co-teacher immediately blushed. The woman realized what she'd done, looked up from the soup, and said, "Well, isn't it okay to moan?" The class cracked up. From then on she was known as "The Moaner."

Kabocha and Butternut Squash Soup with Asian Pear, Apple, and Ginger

The Big O: Apples pop up in so many culinary forms that it's especially important to seek out organic varieties. Scientists at Washington State University conducted a five-year study that showed that organic apples were crisper, tastier, and juicier then their conventionally grown counterparts. Other studies found organic apples are higher in antioxidants. Sounds like a win-win to me!

This is the headliner to my Cashmere Sweater soup collection: It's so soft, cozy, and creamy that your taste buds will know they're feeling the love. The pear, apple, and ginger give this soup layers of flavor.

$^1/_4$ teaspoon ground allspice

$^1/_4$ teaspoon ground cinnamon

$^1/_4$ teaspoon sea salt

$^1/_4$ teaspoon red pepper flakes

$^1/_8$ teaspoon freshly grated nutmeg

2 tablespoons extra virgin olive oil

1 to 2 kabocha squash, halved and seeded

1 butternut squash, halved and seeded

1 cup coarsely chopped yellow onion

1 tablespoon finely chopped shallot

1 teaspoon minced fresh ginger

2 Asian or Anjou pears, peeled, cored, and chopped

1 Rome, Fuji, or McIntosh apple, peeled, cored, and chopped

8 cups Magic Mineral Broth (page 13)

Pomegranate seeds or roasted pumpkin seeds, for garnish

Preheat the oven to 425°F. Line a sheet pan with parchment paper. In a small bowl, whisk the allspice, cinnamon, salt, red pepper flakes, and nutmeg with 1 tablespoon of the olive oil. Brush the inside flesh of the squash with the spice mixture (reserve any remaining) and arrange the squash cut side down on the prepared sheet pan. Roast for 30 minutes, or until very soft. Remove from the oven and let rest until cool.

While the squash is roasting, heat the remaining 1 tablespoon olive oil and the reserved spice mixture in an 8-quart pot over medium heat. Add the onions and a pinch of salt and cook until the onions turn a light golden brown. Add the shallots, sauté for about 3 minutes, and add the ginger, pears, and apples. Continue to sauté for another 3 to 5 minutes, or until the fruit softens and turns golden brown. As the mixture starts to stick to the bottom of the pot, deglaze with 1 cup of the broth. Loosen all the bits from the bottom for great added flavor. Add 3 more cups of the broth and simmer gently.

When the squash has cooled, scoop the flesh into the onion-fruit mixture. Mash the squash mixture with the back of a wooden spoon and add 4 more cups of the broth. Gently simmer for another 15 minutes. Ladle the soup into the blender in small batches and purée until smooth. If the soup is too thick, add more broth. Think FASS: You may want a pinch of salt, a squeeze of lemon, or a few drops of maple syrup. Keep tasting and adjusting to get to Yum! Serve in individual soup bowls, garnished with pomegranate seeds or roasted pumpkin seeds.

Serves 6

PER SERVING Calories: 300; Total Fat: 5 g (1 g saturated, 3 g monounsaturated); Carbohydrates: 64 g; Protein: 7 g; Fiber: 11 g; Sodium: 343 mg

Yukon Gold Potato Leek Soup

I'm fascinated by the concept of fusion cuisine, but it bothers me that it seems limited to Asian and European tastes. I always wanted to apply fusion principles to a traditionally American comfort food, and here it is! Roasted potatoes, roasted garlic, leeks, and rosemary fly together. I'd serve this comfort soup in a colorful bowl; it's earned it.

1 head garlic	1 cup diced yellow onion
3 tablespoons extra virgin olive oil	2 cloves garlic, minced
3 pounds medium Yukon gold potatoes, peeled and chopped	3 leeks, white part only, chopped
1 teaspoon sea salt	8 cups Magic Mineral Broth (page 13) or prepared vegetable or chicken stock
$1/2$ teaspoon freshly ground pepper	Freshly grated nutmeg, for garnish
$1/4$ teaspoon chopped fresh rosemary, or a pinch of dried rosemary	

Preheat the oven to 325°F.

Cut the top off the head of garlic and drizzle with 1 teaspoon of the olive oil. Wrap the garlic in a square of parchment paper and then in a slightly larger piece of aluminum foil. Bake for 45 minutes, or until soft and golden brown. The aroma will tell you when it's ready. Remove from the oven to cool.

Increase the oven temperature to 400°F.

Toss the potatoes with 1 tablespoon of the olive oil, $1/2$ teaspoon salt, the pepper, and rosemary. Spread on a sheet pan and roast for 30 minutes, or until tender. Transfer to a bowl and mash by hand. Set aside.

While the potatoes are roasting, in a 6- to 8-quart pot, heat the remaining olive oil over medium heat. Add the onions and a pinch of salt and sauté for 5 minutes. Add the minced garlic and leeks, decrease the heat, and sauté until both the leeks and the onions are golden. Add the roasted garlic by squeezing it from its skin and sauté for 30 seconds. Deglaze the pot with 1 cup of the stock. Once the liquid evaporates, add 7 cups of the stock and simmer for 15 minutes.

In a blender, purée the potatoes and broth in small batches, adding broth first and then the potatoes; purée until smooth. Return the soup to the pot and taste; you may need to add a pinch of salt or a squeeze of lemon. To serve, ladle the soup into bowls and garnish with a pinch of nutmeg.

Serves 6

PER SERVING Calories: 342; Total Fat: 7 g (1 g saturated, 5 g monounsaturated); Carbohydrates: 61 g; Protein: 8 g; Fiber: 7 g; Sodium: 641 mg

INNER COOK NOTES
You can still make this if you don't have the time or inclination to roast the garlic and the potatoes. Boil the potatoes with a teaspoon of sea salt. When they're tender, drain the water and add a cup of chicken stock or Magic Mineral Broth. Mash well. Add 5 cups of stock. Stir. Add another clove of minced garlic when you sauté the onions and leeks. Pour the potato mixture into the blender, add the leek with rosemary, and blend in batches until it is smooth. Add a little grated nutmeg, taste, and add a pinch of salt if desired.

The Big O: One survey found spuds account for 30 percent of all vegetables consumed in the United States. Imagine my surprise when I found the best of the best at my own farmers' market. Farmer David Little's organic potatoes, pulled straight from Mother Earth, have spoiled me for life. That great taste is part and parcel of how they're raised: on average, organic potatoes are exposed to half the toxins of their commercial brethren. If you do cook with conventionally grown taters, make sure to wash them well and peel them before cooking.

Chicken Stew from My Nana

Most chicken stews are made with a heavy hand; the result is the feeling that you've just consumed dinner for four. My nana knew a better way. This is a much lighter chicken stew, coming in on the gravitational scale somewhere between chicken soup and roast chicken. What makes this dish is both the traditional ingredients and the fact that it simmers as long as a senate filibuster. A little patience pays off in a bountiful stew.

1 whole organic chicken breast, halved, plus 2 drumsticks and 2 thighs

1 teaspoon sea salt

$^1/_2$ teaspoon freshly ground pepper

$^1/_2$ teaspoon plus $^1/_8$ teaspoon paprika

2 tablespoons extra virgin olive oil

2 small yellow onions, cut into bite-size pieces

3 carrots, peeled and cut into bite-size pieces

3 celery stalks, peeled and cut into bite-size pieces

$^1/_4$ teaspoon dried sage

$^1/_4$ teaspoon dried thyme

1 tablespoon minced garlic

4 cups All-Purpose Chicken Stock (page 9)

2 Yukon gold potatoes, peeled and cut into small cubes

Prepare the chicken pieces by rinsing and patting them dry (this will help the chicken brown more evenly). Rub with the salt, pepper, and the $^1/_2$ teaspoon paprika.

In an 8-quart uncovered pot, add the olive oil and heat over medium heat. Add the chicken pieces (you may have to do this in two stages) and brown on both sides. If you begin to lift a piece and it sticks, it's not ready; wait until the chicken lifts easily. Transfer the chicken from the pot to a bowl when both sides are browned.

In the same pot, add half of the onion and one-third of the carrots and celery and sauté until just golden. Add the sage, thyme, garlic, and the $^1/_8$ teaspoon paprika and sauté for 30 seconds. Add 1 cup of the chicken stock to deglaze the pot, using a wooden spoon to scrape all the browned bits from the bottom.

Return the chicken to the pan and add just enough stock to cover, about 3 cups. Simmer for about 45 minutes, or until the chicken is cooked through. Remove the chicken from the stock, cool, and remove the meat from the bone (reserve the bones for No-Fuss Roasted Chicken Stock, page 53). Cut the meat into chunks and add to the broth, along with the potatoes and the remaining onion, carrots, and celery. Simmer until the vegetables are tender, 10 to 15 minutes. Ladle into bowls and serve with crusty bread.

Serves 6

PER SERVING Calories: 433; Total Fat: 13 g (3 g saturated, 6 g monounsaturated); Carbohydrates: 21 g; Protein: 53 g; Fiber: 4 g; Sodium: 758 mg

Lemony Lentil Soup with Pistachio Mint Pesto

My first relationship with lentils began during an apprenticeship at the Chopra Center for Well Being where cooking lentils is a daily ritual. It didn't take long for me to realize these small disks were less time-consuming to prepare than other beans: Lentils cook quickly and require no presoaking. In this recipe, lemon juice adds a bright, light taste, while pesto takes this soup to another level of Yum.

SOUP

2 tablespoons extra virgin olive oil

1 1/2 cups diced yellow onions (about 1 1/2 onions)

Pinches of sea salt

2 carrots, peeled and diced

1 1/2 cups peeled and diced celery

1 tablespoon minced garlic

Pinch to a generous pinch of red pepper flakes

1 teaspoon ground cumin

1 teaspoon ground cinnamon

1/8 teaspoon ground allspice

2 cups green lentils, rinsed well

8 cups Magic Mineral Broth (page 13) or prepared vegetable stock

2 bay leaves

1/2 cup fresh lemon juice

1/4 teaspoon maple syrup

PESTO

1 cup shelled raw pistachios

1/2 cup tightly packed fresh mint leaves

1/4 teaspoon sea salt

1 tablespoon fresh lemon juice

1 tablespoon extra virgin olive oil

INNER COOK NOTES

The pesto can be thinned with a little hot water or stock. Use it as a sauce on pasta or other grains. It's also great with grilled or sautéed vegetables.

The pesto will keep for up to 6 months in the freezer or 1 month in the refrigerator in an airtight container.

Substitute fresh basil for the mint and any nut for the pistachios to create your own pesto combination.

Substitute fennel—which is a good digestive—for celery to add a depth of flavor.

In a large sauté pan, heat the olive oil over medium heat. Add the onions and a pinch of salt and cook until golden brown. Add the carrot, celery, garlic, and red pepper flakes and sauté for about 30 seconds. Add the cumin, cinnamon, allspice, lentils, and a pinch of salt. Stir. Deglaze the pan with 1/2 cup of the broth, letting almost all the liquid evaporate.

Add the remaining 7 1/2 cups broth and the bay leaves. Decrease the heat, cover, and simmer until the vegetables are softened and the lentils have cooked through, about 30 minutes. Taste for doneness after 20 minutes. Add the lemon juice and maple syrup. Taste the soup; you may need to add more lemon juice or a pinch of salt.

To make the pesto, in a food processor fitted with a metal blade, process the pistachios. Add the mint, salt, and lemon juice and process. Drizzle the olive oil through the feed tube and process until smooth, about 2 minutes. Taste. Add a few drops of maple syrup, a pinch of salt, or a few drops of olive oil, if necessary. Ladle the soup into bowls and top with a dollop of pesto.

Serves 6

Although you don't have to presoak lentils, you should rinse them very well. Put lentils in a bowl of cold water and use your hands to swish them around. Drain and repeat the process until the water is clear. As for cooking, don't boil the lentils; that turns them mushy and tends to cause them to fall apart. Let the lentils simmer for a nice, tender texture.

PER SERVING Calories: 467; Total Fat: 18 g (2 g saturated, 10 g monounsaturated); Carbohydrates: 59 g; Protein: 19 g; Fiber: 16 g; Sodium: 392 mg

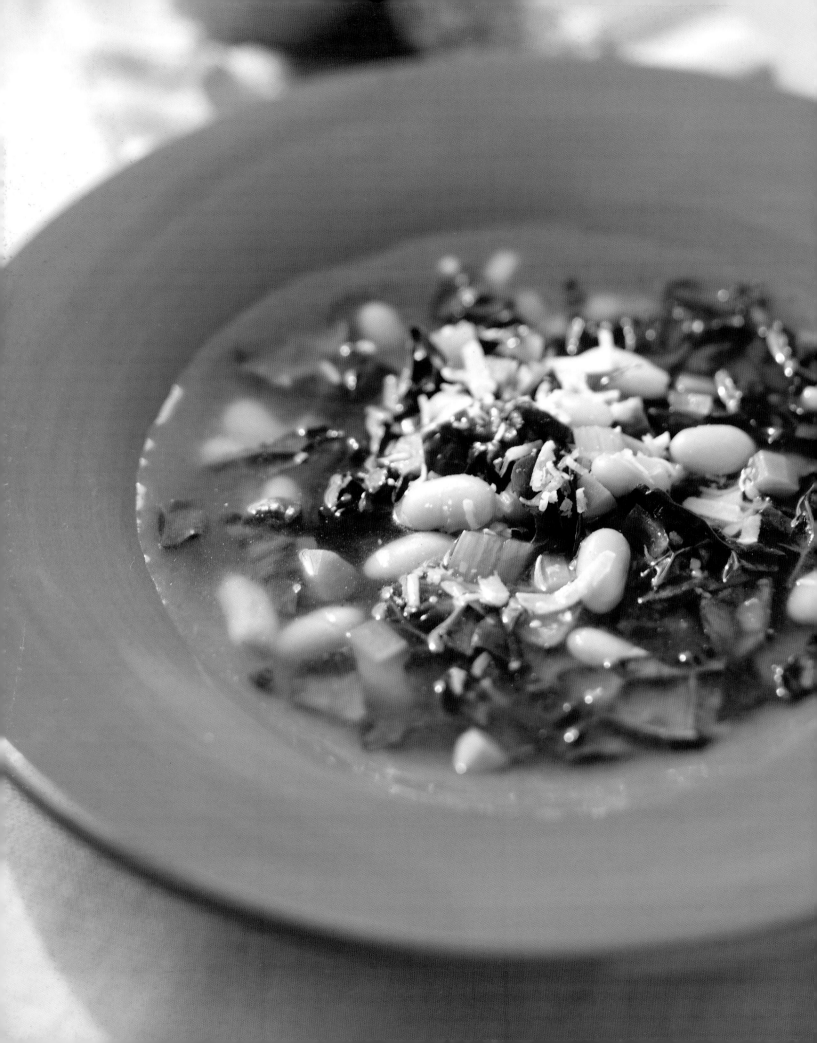

Tuscan Bean Soup with Kale

White Italian kidney beans make a delicious, hearty base for a soup. Add a dollop of pesto and some freshly grated Parmesan and I personally guarantee that everyone at the table will melt before your eyes.

BEANS

2 cups presoaked cannellini or great Northern white beans (page 150)

2 sprigs fresh rosemary, or $1/4$ teaspoon dried rosemary

$1/8$ teaspoon dried sage, or $1/4$ teaspoon fresh sage

2 sprigs fresh thyme, or $1/4$ teaspoon dried thyme

4 cloves garlic, smashed

SOUP

2 tablespoons extra virgin olive oil

$1^3/4$ cups finely chopped yellow onion

$1^1/2$ cups peeled and diced carrots

$1^1/2$ cups peeled and diced celery

1 tablespoon diced shallot

$1/4$ teaspoon sea salt

2 tablespoons finely chopped garlic

$1/4$ teaspoon fresh thyme, or $1/8$ teaspoon dried thyme

$1/8$ teaspoon fresh sage, or a pinch of dried sage

$1/8$ teaspoon fresh oregano, or a pinch of dried oregano

8 cups Magic Mineral Broth (page 13)

1 bunch of dino kale or Swiss chard, stemmed and chopped into small bite-size pieces

A dollop of pesto (page 115) and a sprinkle of organic Parmesan cheese, for serving

Cook the beans following the method on page 150, adding a sachet of rosemary, sage, thyme, and garlic to the cooking liquid.

In an 8-quart pot, heat the olive oil over medium-high heat. Add the onions and a pinch of salt. Sauté until golden. Add the carrots, celery, shallot, and $1/4$ teaspoon salt. Sauté for 3 minutes more. Add the garlic, thyme, sage, and oregano and sauté for 2 minutes more.

Deglaze the pot with $1/4$ cup of the broth. Allow the liquid to evaporate. Add 6 cups more broth, and the beans, and simmer for 20 minutes. Add more broth if necessary to achieve the desired consistency. Add the greens and a pinch of salt and simmer until the greens have wilted. Think FASS: You may need to add a squeeze of lemon juice or a final pinch of salt. Serve in soup bowls with a dollop of pesto and a sprinkle of Parmesan cheese.

Serves 6

PER SERVING Calories: 410; Total Fat: 10 g (1 g saturated, 7 g monounsaturated); Carbohydrates: 59 g; Protein: 18 g; Fiber: 15 g; Sodium: 449 mg

INNER COOK NOTES

To save time use canned organic cannellini beans. Remember to give them a rinse and a squeeze of lemon and a pinch of salt to freshen them up. For a seasonal twist, add diced delicata squash to the carrot, celery, and onion mixture.

Some clients like to eat, and some don't. One person I cook for hated food long before he became sick. If he could eat a pill instead of food, he would do it. The few foods he enjoyed were connected with his travels to Italy and Japan. When we did our initial interview, he mentioned that he liked baked beans as a kid. I figured if he liked beans and loved Italy, he might enjoy this dish. His reaction? A bowl of soup he looked forward to eating! As he put it, "This soup tastes too good to be healthy."

You can use any type of kale for this recipe. Just make sure it's cut into small bite-size pieces so it stays on your spoon and is easy to digest.

Black Bean Chili

One time I was in a rush making this dish, which led to a serendipitous discovery. With no time to soak beans, I grabbed a can of cooked organic beans. Not a bad backup, and quick to boot. Here's how you bring out their taste: Rinse the beans and squeeze a little lemon or lime juice over them. Then add 1/8 teaspoon sea salt. After they've been asleep in the can, wake them up with this spa treatment.

The Big O: When it comes to peppers, good things come in small packages. While commercially grown peppers are flooded with nitrogen to make them grow larger, those behemoths tend to be taste challenged. Think of adding a teaspoon of honey to your tea versus your stockpot, and you'll get the idea. Organic peppers, while smaller, are far tastier and more nutrient-dense, with all their powerful antioxidants in place. Think of it: A healing chili! Now there's a concept.

That's right, chili. Sky-high, make you slap your thighs, as hot or as cool as you like it chili. Surprised? Me, too. I couldn't imagine anyone going through chemo wanting chili, but that only shows you what I know. I've cooked for some folks who, when the urge hits them, want their chili now! I make sure they have it, in a way that won't do a number on their often delicate tummies. One key is using red and yellow peppers, which, unlike green peppers, are sweet, nutritious, and easy to stomach. I realized this dish had more than enough flavor when I once forgot the chili powder and no one noticed. Still, you can use the chili powder to run up the alarms.

2 tablespoons extra virgin olive oil

1 cup chopped yellow onion

Pinches of sea salt

1 1/2 cups chopped red, orange, and yellow bell peppers (small bite-size pieces)

3 cloves garlic, minced

1 fresh jalapeño pepper, ribs and seeds removed, finely chopped

0 to 3 tablespoons chili powder (based on your taste buds!)

1 teaspoon ground cumin

1 teaspoon dried oregano

1/2 teaspoon ground cinnamon

1 (28-ounce) can crushed tomatoes

1/2 teaspoon rapadura or other organic sweetener (optional)

2 (15-ounce) cans organic black beans, drained, rinsed, and mixed with a spritz of fresh lemon juice and a pinch of salt, or 4 cups cooked from dried (page 150)

Avocado Cream (page 115) (optional)

In a 6-quart pot, heat the olive oil over medium heat. Add the onions and a pinch of salt and sauté for 3 minutes, until soft. Add the bell peppers and sauté until just tender. Add the garlic and jalapeño pepper and sauté for 30 seconds.

Stir in chili powder to taste, the cumin, oregano, and cinnamon. Mix thoroughly to coat the onions and peppers. Stir in the tomatoes, a pinch of salt, rapadura, and 1 cup of water. Cover and bring to a boil. Decrease the heat and simmer for 20 minutes. Remove the lid, add the beans and a pinch of salt, and simmer, uncovered, for about 15 minutes, stirring occasionally.

Serve in individual bowls garnished with a dollop of Avocado Cream.

Serves 6

PER SERVING Calories: 237; Total Fat: 5 g (0 g saturated, 3 g monounsaturated); Carbohydrates: 39 g; Protein: 12 g; Fiber: 14 g; Sodium: 771 mg

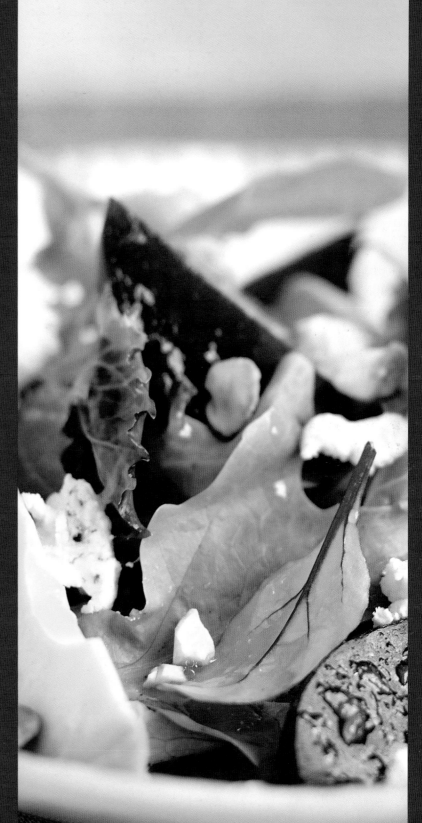

If you grew up like I did, you probably couldn't imagine enjoying vegetables. I remember my mom treating vegetables like they were castor oil: good for me (perhaps) but drowned in invocations of dread: "Rebecca Irene Katz, you are not getting up from the table until you eat your vegetables!"

NOW, MY MOM WASN'T BAD WITH VEGETABLES. They weren't the gray, bland mush some of my friends and clients were raised on. Even so, many a broccoli spear got slipped to my dog. Once I put my veggies in an envelope and addressed it to my mother's favorite culinary charity, "The Starving Children of China." My friend's mom tried hiding spinach in one of his favorite foods, mashed potatoes. His reaction? "Yuck."

All these years later and Mom's voice has been replaced by the nutritionist's: "Don't just eat your vegetables. *Eat five servings a day.*" You think, "I'd rather have the castor oil."

Yet, you also know the nutritionist is right. Veggies—especially crunchy green, yellow, orange, and cruciferous vegetables—contain all the phyto-chemicals, antioxidants, vitamins, and minerals we need to maintain health. Many have been shown to help lower the risk of certain cancers.

So how do you make these fearful cruciferi taste, smell, and look great? That's what the recipes in this chapter are all about. They're designed to take you from that place of "I *have* to eat my vegetables," to "I *want* to eat my vegetables because they're yummy!"

The first step is preparation: This means looking beyond your vegetable steamer. Steaming is fine, but after a while steaming gets pretty boring. Then you give up eating your veggies. No veggies means no nutrition. I want to keep your interest in vegetables piqued. Roasting, sautéing, stir-frying, puréeing, and baking: there are lots of ways to bring out the maximum flavor and nutritional value of vegetables so that you'll eat them. Also, some people with cancer find raw vegetables hard to digest. Cooking vegetables with the spices and other ingredients we've chosen releases their scrumptious taste while making them easier on the tummy.

Step two is using organic produce whenever possible (which I hope is all the time). Hang around a farmers' market for a bit and you'll also learn when different vegetables are at the height of their season, ready for the table.

The final step is what I call shaking it up, or the culinary equivalent of accessorizing. A staple such as the string bean takes on a whole new look and taste when dressed up with a little feta cheese and cherry tomatoes. Broccoli is no longer boring when it's quickly blanched and then sautéed in olive oil and garlic or ginger. Squash, kale, and yes, even spinach: you'll be astounded how a little prep and creativity can take these vegetables from onerous to outstanding in just a few minutes. I'll even show you how to go Mom one better, by deliciously hiding vegetables in places that no one would suspect, such as tarts and pizza crusts. One bite and there will be plenty of veggie converts.

Baby Bok Choy with Sesame and Ginger

Sometimes I just love the name of a food, the way the sound rolls off my tongue. Bok choy. Say it with me three times fast: bok choy, bok choy, bok choy! It sounds so exotic that if you can make it, you must be a pretty good cook. Bok choy is Asian cabbage, a staple in Chinese cuisine. It's also a cruciferous vegetable. That means it's very, very, very good for you. Bok choy's flavor is naturally pungent; the sesame and ginger in this recipe temper it beautifully.

INNER COOK NOTES
The ingredients list looks long, but the prep time is short. The short cooking time is what keeps the bok choy crisp.

4 to 6 heads baby bok choy (about 1 pound)

1¹/₂ tablespoons brown rice vinegar

1¹/₂ tablespoons tamari

1 tablespoon mirin

¹/₂ teaspoon maple syrup

1 teaspoon toasted sesame oil

1 tablespoon sesame oil

Pinch of red pepper flakes

2 medium cloves garlic, minced

1 tablespoon minced fresh ginger root

2 scallions, both white and green parts, sliced

Squeeze of fresh lime juice

1 tablespoon toasted sesame seeds (see page 151)

Trim the bases off the bok choy heads. Separate the bok choy into individual leaves and cut crosswise into bite-size pieces, keeping the stems and leaves separate.

Combine the vinegar, tamari, mirin, maple syrup, and toasted sesame oil in a bowl, and set aside.

Stir-frying is very fast, so have everything ready to go.

Preheat a wok or sauté pan over high heat, add the sesame oil, and swirl to glaze the pan. Add the bok choy stems, red pepper flakes, garlic, ginger, and scallions. Stir-fry for 30 seconds.

Add the sauce mixture and cook until thickened, about 1 minute. Add the bok choy leaves and continue to cook for another 30 seconds, until the bok choy is just wilted.

Transfer the bok choy to a serving bowl, add a squeeze of lime, and sprinkle with the sesame seeds. Serve immediately.

Serves 4

PER SERVING Calories: 96; Total Fat: 7 g (0 g saturated, 2 g monounsaturated); Carbohydrates: 6 g; Protein: 3 g; Fiber: 2 g; Sodium: 225 mg

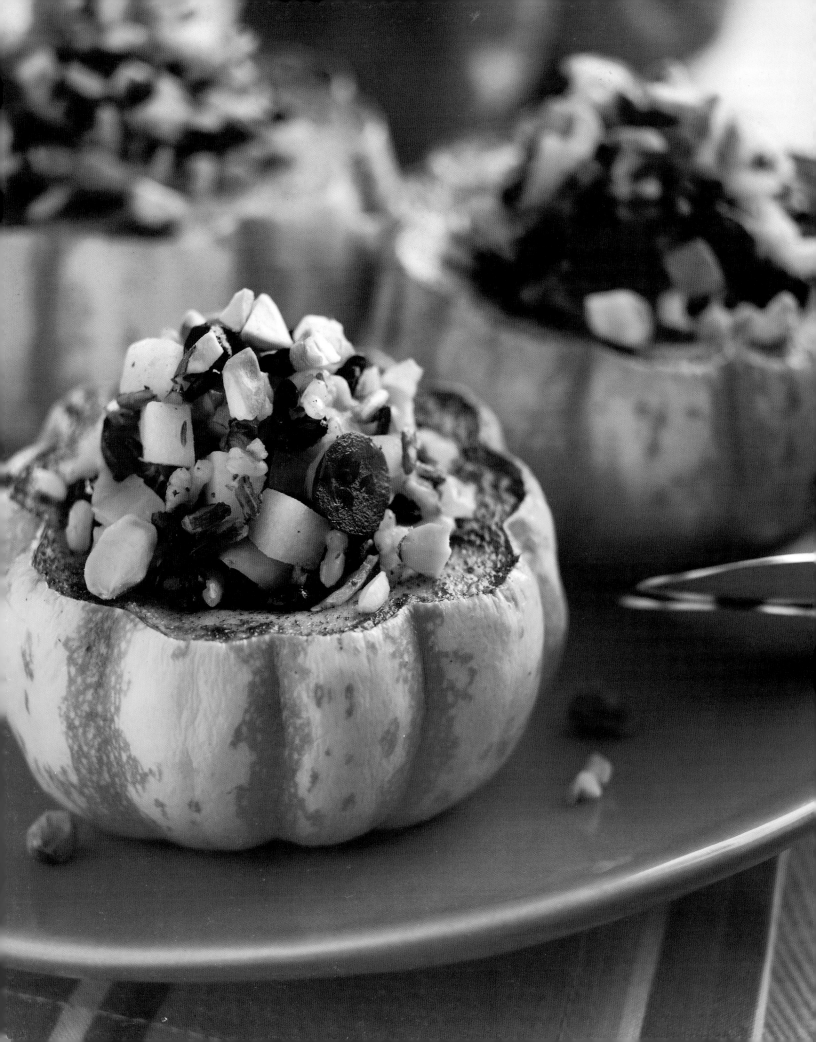

Baby Dumpling Squash Stuffed with Rice Medley

Everybody has their cue that fall has arrived. The kids go back to school. The leaves turn vivid colors, and the NFL creates couch potatoes. For me, the tip-off that the autumnal equinox is at hand is that baby dumpling squash has made their return to the farmers' market. When cut in half across its girth, the squash turns into its own individual serving bowl ready to be filled with rice, veggies, or just about any type of grain. To score a perfect ten, concentrate on bringing out the squash's home-grown sweet flavor and finding a stuffing that's visually appealing. This is one of those dishes that, once put together, looks too pretty to eat. The squash resembles a miniature yellow pumpkin laced with orange and green stripes. Take a moment for art appreciation, then dive in and experience an explosion of flavor.

SQUASH

1 tablespoon extra virgin olive oil

$1/4$ teaspoon sea salt

$1/4$ teaspoon ground allspice

$1/4$ teaspoon red pepper flakes

$1/4$ teaspoon ground cinnamon

6 to 8 baby dumpling squash, tops cut off, center and seeds scooped out

RICE MEDLEY

1 cup Lundberg brown and wild rice blend

1 cup Emporia's Forbidden Rice or Lundberg Japonica Rice

1 teaspoon sea salt

2 tablespoons extra virgin olive oil

1 cup diced yellow onion

1 cup peeled and diced celery

2 tablespoons finely chopped shallots

2 pippin, Granny Smith, or Fuji apples, peeled, cored, and cut into small cubes

$1/4$ teaspoon dried thyme

$1/4$ teaspoon dried sage

$1/2$ cup dried cranberries, currants, or raisins

1 cup chopped roasted pistachios (see page 151) (optional)

A little prep here goes a long way. Roast the squash in advance and make the rice a day ahead of time (by the way, you can add a cup of lentils to the rice mix if you want some extra protein). For smaller gatherings, the recipe can easily be halved. You can also reheat leftovers by placing the stuffed squash in a covered baking dish. Reheat at 350°F for 15 minutes, or until the squash is warmed throughout.

Preheat the oven to 350°F. Line a rimmed sheet pan with parchment paper. Combine the olive oil, salt, allspice, red pepper flakes, and cinnamon. Brush the insides of the squash with the spice mixture. Arrange the squash cut side down on the prepared sheet pan and roast for 20 to 25 minutes, or until tender. Check them at 20 minutes, touching the top of a squash with your finger. If they're soft, remove them from the oven and cover with foil until ready for assembly.

To make the rice medley, in two saucepans bring 2 cups of water in each to a boil with $1/2$ teaspoon salt in each pan. Add one type of rice to each pan, return to a boil, cover, and decrease the heat to low. Simmer until tender, about 30 minutes. Transfer both types of rice to one sheet pan and rake with a fork to separate the grains.

(continued on next page)

While the rice is cooking, heat 2 tablespoons olive oil in a sauté pan. Add the onion with a pinch of salt and sauté for about 5 minutes, until golden. Add the celery, shallot, and apples and sauté for another 3 minutes. Add the thyme, sage, and cranberries and sauté for 2 minutes more. Deglaze the pan with 2 tablespoons water.

In a large bowl, combine the vegetable-apple mixture with the rice. Think FASS: Taste the mixture; you may need to add a pinch or two of salt.

To assemble the dish, scoop the rice mixture into the squashes. Serve each squash topped with a sprinkling of the toasted pistachios. Serve all on a platter or individual plates as a main dish.

Serves 6

PER SERVING Calories: 427; Total Fat: 9 g (1 g saturated, 5 g monounsaturated); Carbohydrates: 84 g; Protein: 9 g; Fiber: 9 g; Sodium: 512 mg

Broccoli Sautéed with Garlic

With all due respect to a former president, you need to eat your broccoli. It's an absolute stud vegetable, abundantly rich in immunity-building phytochemicals. That said, broccoli can get awfully boring when it's served day after day in a steaming heap. To keep you from becoming broccoli-challenged, consider this recipe with a Mediterranean twist.

$^1/_2$ teaspoon sea salt	1 tablespoon extra virgin olive oil
1 large bunch broccoli, cut into florets, stems peeled, and cut into bite-size pieces	1 tablespoon chopped garlic
	Pinch of red pepper flakes

Bring a large pot of water to a boil. Add the $^1/_2$ teaspoon salt. Blanch the broccoli for 30 seconds. Transfer with a slotted spoon to a cold water bath so that the broccoli retains its lush green color.

In a medium sauté pan, heat the olive oil over medium-high heat. Add the garlic and red pepper flakes and sauté for 30 seconds, just until aromatic. Add the broccoli and a pinch of salt and sauté for 2 minutes. The broccoli will be al dente.

Serve hot or at room temperature.

Serves 4

PER SERVING Calories: 70; Total Fat: 4 g (0 g saturated, 2 g monounsaturated); Carbohydrates: 6 g; Protein: 2 g; Fiber: 2 g; Sodium: 323 mg

INNER COOK NOTES
For a variation, add 1 teaspoon finely grated fresh ginger to the garlic and red pepper flakes. For a more Mediterranean dish, top the broccoli with pine nuts, caramelized onions, and currants.

Don't toss the stalk when cooking broccoli: Use it; it's sweet and nutritious. To speed up prep time, broccoli can be blanched and shocked and then stored in an airtight container in the fridge. Sautéing it when you're ready to eat takes only minutes.

Szechwan Broccoli

In this recipe we go a step beyond steaming; sautéed broccoli retains all its nutrients, which may come as a surprise (and a relief) to those who believe that only raw broccoli is nutritious. Szechwan Broccoli, as the name implies, is Asian fare.

2 bunches broccoli

$1/2$ teaspoon sea salt

2 tablespoons brown rice vinegar

2 tablespoons tamari

1 tablespoon mirin

$1/2$ teaspoon toasted sesame oil

1 teaspoon maple syrup

2 teaspoons sesame oil

Pinch of red pepper flakes or cayenne

3 cloves garlic, minced

1 tablespoon minced fresh ginger

2 scallions, both green and white parts, minced

INNER COOK NOTES
For a change of pace, top with cashews or Pecans Spiced with Orange Zest and Ginger (page 95).

Remove the florets from the broccoli. Peel the broccoli stems with a vegetable peeler until smooth. Slice the stems into bite-size pieces.

Bring a large pot of water to a boil. Add the salt. Add the broccoli and blanch for 30 seconds. Transfer with a slotted spoon to a cold water bath to stop the cooking and preserve the broccoli's color. Drain the broccoli and set aside.

In a small bowl mix the vinegar, tamari, mirin, toasted sesame oil, and maple syrup.

Have all your ingredients ready for a quick finish. Heat a wok or sauté pan over medium-high heat. Add the sesame oil, red pepper flakes, garlic, ginger, and scallions. Stir quickly for about 30 seconds, just until aromatic.

Add the sauce to the wok and simmer until thickened, about 30 seconds. Add the broccoli and heat through, about 15 seconds. Serve immediately.

Serves 6

PER SERVING Calories: 76; Total Fat: 2 g (0 g saturated, 1 g monounsaturated); Carbohydrates: 11 g; Protein: 4 g; Fiber: 3 g; Sodium: 365 mg

Dark Leafy Greens with Caramelized Onions, Raisins, and Pine Nuts

One trick to preparing greens is ripping them off their tough spines. This makes them easier to eat and digest. Once you've stemmed your greens (a great job for the little ones), chop them (the greens, not the kids) into bite-size pieces with your sharp chef's knife. When you add your greens to the pan, they will resemble Mount Vesuvius, but you'll be surprised how quickly that volcano of greens shrinks into a small mound.

Another trick for preparing greens is to put them in a bowl of cold water for a bath; this allows dirt and sand to fall to the bottom. Remove the greens from the water, roll the leaves in bunches, cut them into thin ribbons, and then cut length-wise into small bite-size pieces.

Most people I know are intimidated by dark leafy greens. They buy them because they should, yet the greens always seem to end up either in a vase as a bouquet or permanently exiled to the hinterlands of the fridge. Here's a better solution: adding a few raisins and caramelized onions cuts the bitterness of the greens by introducing some sweetness. My friend said her four-year-old ate these greens and said they tasted like candy. That's a kid with a bright future.

6 cups kale or Swiss chard, stemmed, and cut into bite-size pieces

2 tablespoons extra virgin olive oil

1 red onion, cut into quarter moons (about 1 cup)

Pinch of sea salt

1 clove garlic, minced

1/3 cup raisins or currants

1 tablespoon toasted pine nuts (see page 151) (optional)

Cover the kale with cold water and set aside until ready to use.

In a large, deep sauté pan, heat the olive oil over medium-high heat. Add the onions and a pinch of salt. Sauté for 3 to 5 minutes. Decrease the heat to low and cook slowly until the onions are caramelized, about 20 minutes.

Add the garlic and stir for about 30 seconds, just until aromatic. Add the raisins and stir for about 30 seconds. Deglaze the pan with 2 tablespoons of water to loosen all the flavorful bits from the bottom.

Begin adding the greens to the pan with a pinch of salt, continuing to add as many greens as will fit in the pan.

The water that adheres to the greens will be enough liquid to wilt the greens. Taste the greens, add an additional tablespoon of water, if needed, cover the pan, and cook the greens until tender, 2 to 3 minutes. Taste again, adding of pinch of salt or a drop or two of maple syrup, if necessary.

Arrange the greens on a plate and sprinkle with the toasted pine nuts. Serve hot. Don't forget to pour the cooking juices over the greens before you add the nuts—more nutrients!

Serves 6

PER SERVING Calories: 109; Total Fat: 5 g (1 g saturated, 3 g monounsaturated); Carbohydrates: 15 g; Protein: 3 g; Fiber: 2 g; Sodium: 129 mg

Garlicky Leafy Greens

For more information on greens, see the note on page 36.

2 bunches tender kale, Swiss chard, or spinach (about 6 cups)

1 tablespoon extra virgin olive oil

2 cloves garlic, minced

Pinch of red pepper flakes

$1/_4$ teaspoon sea salt

Squeeze of fresh lemon juice

Remove all tough stems from the greens, chop the greens into bite-size pieces, and cover with cold water. Set aside.

In a medium sauté pan, heat the olive oil over medium-high heat. Add the garlic and red pepper flakes and sauté for 30 seconds, just until aromatic. Add the greens and salt and sauté until the greens begin to darken and intensify.

If necessary, add a splash of water to cook the greens until they're tender. Add the lemon juice and taste the greens. You may need to add a pinch of salt or a few drops of maple syrup to round out the flavor. Serve immediately on a small platter.

Makes about 2 cups (Serves 4)

PER SERVING Calories: 83; Total Fat: 4 g (1 g saturated, 3 g monounsaturated); Carbohydrates: 11 g; Protein: 3 g; Fiber: 2 g; Sodium: 191 mg

Jicama and Red Cabbage Salad with Mint and Cilantro Tossed with Sweet-and-Sour Asian Dressing

A friend of mine was laid up in bed one summer with a serious illness. This woman goes nuts if she's in the house for two days; now she was facing a six-week convalescence. On the second day, I called her to see if she wanted some food. "I'm climbing the walls and feel like a caged animal. I need some 'outside' in; I want that feeling of outdoors in me." I went over and made this salad. After that, this dish is all she wanted for the next month. Even now, she says, "If I feel punky, I make this salad."

If you're a coleslaw fan or have a jones for a crunchy salad, this recipe is for you. Red cabbage is a nutrient-rich cruciferous vegetable. Jicama is loaded with nutrients, including iron. Together they make a colorful pair. This salad goes well with fish and turkey burgers or the Miso Salmon with Lime-Ginger Glaze (page 60).

NUTS

$^1/_2$ cup sliced almonds

1 tablespoon maple syrup

Pinch of cayenne

DRESSING

$^1/_2$ teaspoon seeded and diced jalapeño

3 tablespoons rice vinegar

1 tablespoon fresh lime juice

$^1/_4$ cup tamari

3 tablespoons maple syrup

1 teaspoon toasted sesame oil

1 tablespoon minced fresh ginger

Pinch of sea salt

SALAD

1 pound red cabbage (about 6 cups chopped)

$^1/_2$ pound jicama, peeled, small julienned (about 4 cups)

2 tablespoons finely chopped fresh mint

$^1/_4$ cup finely chopped fresh cilantro or fresh basil

Preheat the oven to 350°F.

Toss the nuts in a bowl with the maple syrup and cayenne. Spread on a sheet pan and bake for 10 to 12 minutes, until golden and fragrant. Remove from the oven and cool to room temperature. Use a metal spatula to loosen the crispy nuts.

To make the dressing, whisk together the jalapeño, vinegar, lime juice, tamari, maple syrup, sesame oil, ginger, and salt. Set aside.

To make the salad, cut the cabbage in half, remove the core, and shred with a sharp knife.

In a large bowl, combine the cabbage, jicama, mint, and cilantro. Toss with the dressing. Sprinkle the nuts on top and serve.

Serves 6

PER SERVING Calories: 131; Total Fat: 5 g (0 g saturated, 3 g monounsaturated); Carbohydrates: 19 g; Protein: 5 g; Fiber: 5 g; Sodium: 336 mg

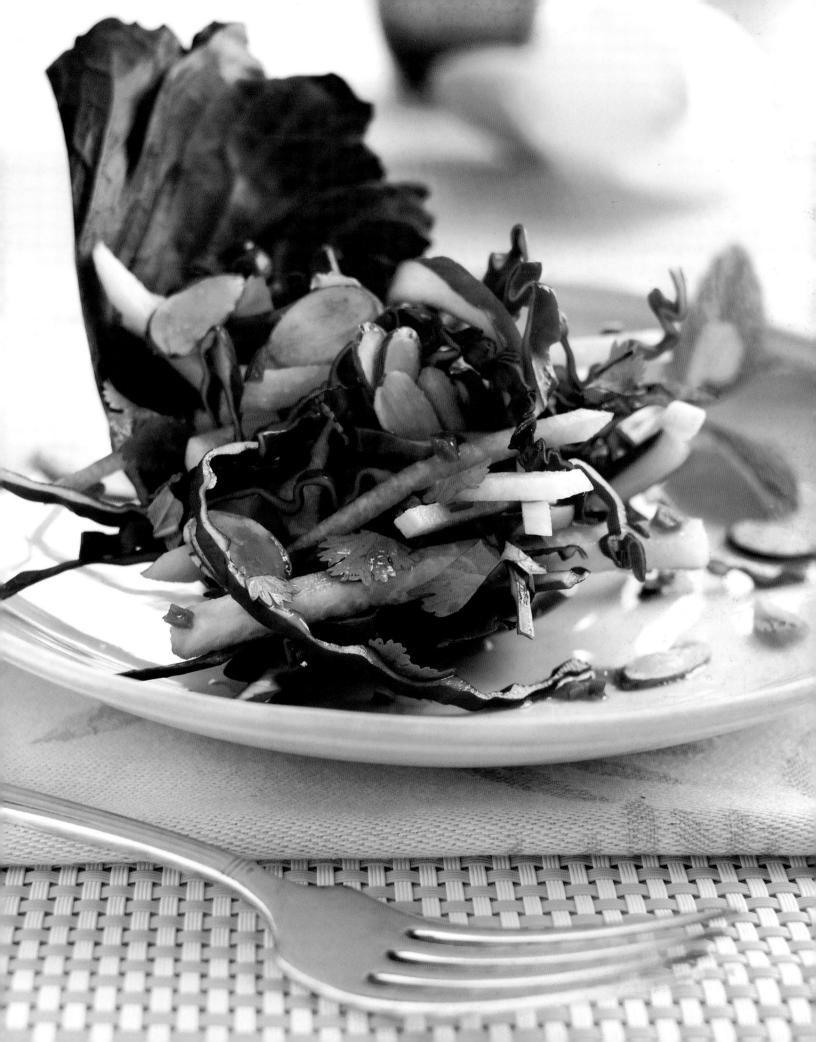

Swiss Chard Braised with Sweet Tomatoes and Corn

For more information on greens, see the note on page 36.

1 bunch Swiss chard or dino kale, stemmed and chopped into small pieces

2 tablespoons extra virgin olive oil

1 teaspoon minced garlic

$1/_8$ teaspoon red pepper flakes

Pinches of sea salt

1 cup cooked corn kernals

24 sungold tomatoes or a mix of cherry and small pear-shaped tomatoes, halved

Cover the Swiss chard with cold water and set aside until ready to use.

Heat the olive oil in a large sauté pan over medium-high heat. Add the garlic, red pepper flakes, and a pinch of salt. Sauté for 30 seconds, just until aromatic.

Add the greens and a pinch of salt and sauté until wilted. The soaking water that adheres to the greens will help wilt and cook the greens.

Add the corn and tomatoes and cook for another 2 to 3 minutes, or until tender. Taste for doneness.

Serve immediately in a small serving bowl. The colors brighten any table.

Serves 4

PER SERVING Calories: 298; Total Fat: 10 g (1 g saturated, 6 g monounsaturated); Carbohydrates: 48 g; Protein: 14 g; Fiber: 10 g; Sodium: 425 mg

Delicata Squash with Dino Kale and Cranberries

This is another recipe that shows FASS in action. Alone, these veggies might prove overwhelming, especially for people with sensitive taste buds or stomachs. Together, their flavors make a magnificent, balanced blend. The fat comes from olive oil, the sweet from the squash. These two ingredients balance the slightly pungent taste of kale and the eye-popping tartness of cranberry. I came up with this recipe while humming to a llama. Really. The restaurant I used to work in had an organic garden and a llama sanctuary attached to it. I was musing to Alfred (he's the llama; they communicate by humming), wondering what to do with all the autumn squash and kale that was being harvested from the garden. The next thing I knew, I'd come up with the dish and put it on the menu. When they flew out the door, we knew we had a hit on our hands. The next time I saw Alfred, he hummed to me that I owed him a commission.

INNER COOK NOTES
This mixture can be used to fill individual galettes (page 87).

This makes a wonderful side dish. It can also be served as a main course tossed with noodles or served over Garlicky Brown Basmati Rice (page 89).

6 cups dino kale, stemmed and torn into small bite-size pieces

4 delicata squash

2 tablespoons extra virgin olive oil

$1/4$ teaspoon dried sage

$1/4$ teaspoon ground allspice

$1/2$ teaspoon sea salt

$1/8$ teaspoon red pepper flakes

$1/4$ cup dried cranberries

Preheat the oven to 425°F.

Cover the kale with cold water and set aside until ready to use.

Peel the squash with a sharp vegetable peeler. Cut in half lengthwise, scoop out the core and seeds, and cut into $1/2$-inch pieces. Toss the squash with 1 tablespoon of the olive oil, the sage, allspice, and $1/4$ teaspoon of the salt. Spread the squash in a single layer on a baking sheet. Roast for 15 minutes, or until tender.

While the squash is roasting, heat a large sauté pan over medium heat. Add the remaining 1 tablespoon olive oil, the red pepper flakes, and cranberries. Stir for 10 seconds and add the kale and the remaining $1/4$ teaspoon salt. Sauté until tender. The water that adheres to the greens should be enough water to cook the greens. If needed, add 1 tablespoon water to finish cooking.

Stir the roasted squash into the sautéed kale. Serve immediately in a shallow serving bowl or as a side dish to a main course.

Serves 4

PER SERVING Calories: 298; Total Fat: 8 g (1 g saturated, 5 g monounsaturated); Carbohydrates: 57 g; Protein: 8 g; Fiber: 10 g; Sodium: 357 mg

Mixed Greens with Roasted Beets and Avocado Tossed with Orange-Shallot Vinaigrette

This beautiful salad represents a harmonic convergence of tastes. The spiciness of some of the greens in a spring mix is balanced by the avocado's creamy, healthy fat, while the sweetness of the roasted beets cuts the acidic nature of the citrus dressing.

INNER COOK NOTES

If the beets vary in size, wrap them accordingly so you can remove the package of smaller ones when tender, leaving the larger ones in the oven until they are tender.

Removing the beet skins can be messy work. To lessen the mess, transfer the beets directly from the oven to a plastic bag to steam until they can be handled easily. The skins will come right off. Wear gloves, or use the plastic bag to protect your hands from turning beet red.

3 medium or 5 small beets (1 to 1¼ cups small cubes), trimmed and washed

DRESSING

2 cups organic fresh squeezed orange juice

1 tablespoon diced shallot

2 tablespoons extra virgin olive oil

1½ tablespoons fresh lemon juice

¼ teaspoon sea salt

¼ teaspoon maple syrup (optional)

1 Hass avocado, thinly sliced

Squeeze of fresh lemon or lime juice

6 to 8 cups mixed salad greens, rinsed and spun dry

5 ounces organic goat cheese, crumbled (optional)

⅓ cup chopped pistachios or other nuts, toasted (see page 151) (optional)

Preheat the oven to 425°F. Wrap the beets in parchment paper, then in foil, and roast for 30 minutes to 1 hour (depending on size), until tender and fragrant. Remove from the oven, cool, and peel. Cut into small cubes, thin slices, or julienne.

While the beets are roasting, make the dressing. Bring the orange juice and shallots to a boil over high heat in a sauté pan. Decrease the heat to medium and simmer until the liquid has reduced by half (about 20 minutes, but it could happen faster, so don't wander too far). Remove from the heat and cool to room temperature.

Slowly whisk the oil, lemon juice, and sea salt into the orange juice. Taste the dressing; you may need a spritz of lemon juice, a pinch of salt, or a few drops of maple syrup.

To assemble the salad, toss the avocado slices with the lemon juice to prevent them from browning. In a large bowl, combine the greens, avocado, and beets. Coat lightly with the dressing. Arrange the salad on a plate and top with the goat cheese and toasted pistachios.

Serves 6

PER SERVING Calories: 148; Total Fat: 9 g (1 g saturated, 6 g monounsaturated); Carbohydrates: 17 g; Protein: 2 g; Fiber: 4 g; Sodium: 140 mg

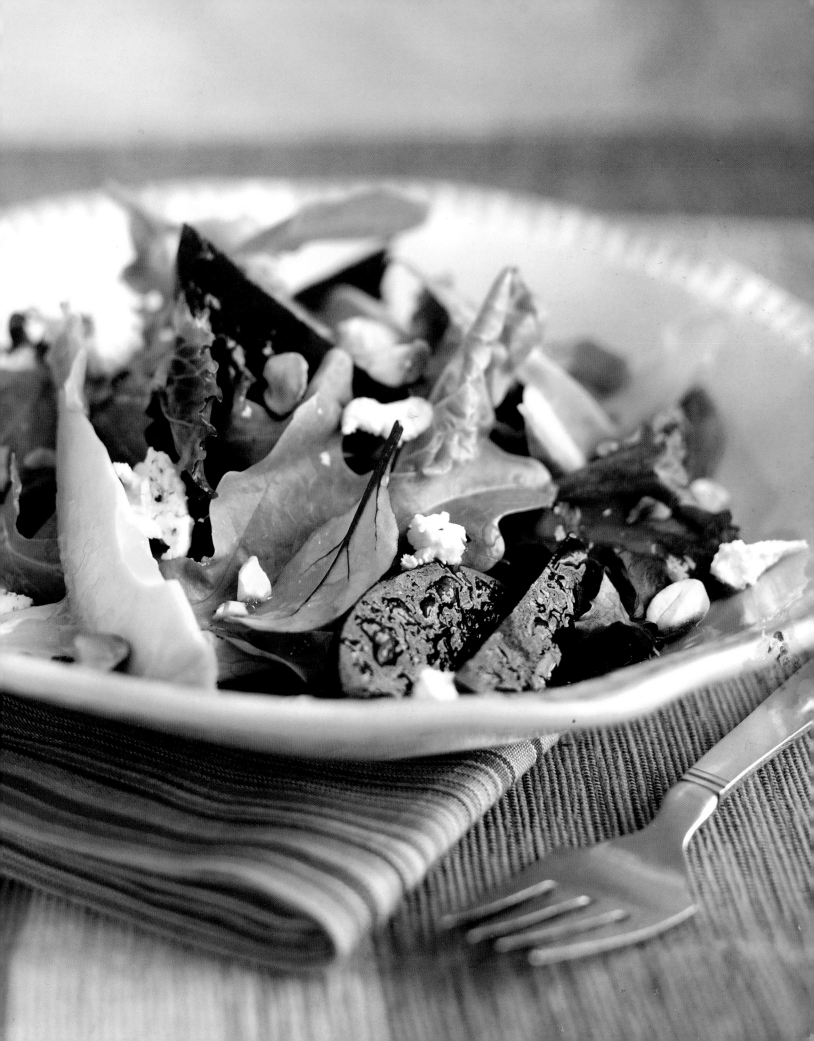

My Favorite Salad with Bright Mediterranean Vinaigrette

INNER COOK NOTES
This dish is best in summer, when tomatoes are in season. If you don't like tomatoes, you can leave them out. It's still an excellent salad.

The Big O: Of all the veggies out there, organic lettuce is the easiest to find because it's so easy to grow. Supermarkets and farmers' markets abound with numerous varieties of organic lettuce. Conventionally grown lettuce, as you might guess, is highly susceptible to the high levels of chemicals it usually receives.

I love this salad. I dream about this salad. It's a variation on fattoush, *a fabulously named Mediterranean salad. This is the freshest, cleanest salad I can imagine. It's like Nautilus for the taste buds: the sweetness of fresh tomatoes, a starburst of fresh mint and parsley, creamy cheese, salty olives, crispy pita chips, and crunchy lettuce . . . like I said, it's a workout for the palate. Like most workouts, you'll feel wonderful after you eat it.*

2 pitas

DRESSING

$1^1/_2$ tablespoons fresh lemon juice

$^1/_4$ cup extra virgin olive oil

1 teaspoon brown rice vinegar

$^1/_4$ teaspoon ground cumin

$^1/_4$ teaspoon sea salt

SALAD

6 to 8 cups romaine hearts, roughly chopped

1 English cucumber, peeled, seeded, and cut into small pieces

1 pint cherry tomatoes, halved

3 to 4 ounces organic feta cheese

1 cup kalamata olives, pitted and halved lengthwise

$^1/_4$ cup chopped fresh mint

$^1/_4$ cup chopped fresh flat-leaf parsley

Preheat the oven to 350°F. Cut the pitas into quarters, split into layers, and place on a sheet pan. Bake for 8 to 10 minutes, until golden. Remove from the oven and cool. Break the baked pitas into small pieces and set aside.

To make the dressing, combine the lemon juice, olive oil, vinegar, cumin, and salt in a small bowl. Whisk to incorporate. Set aside until ready to use.

In a large salad bowl, toss the romaine hearts with the dressing. Top with the cucumber, tomatoes, feta, and olives. Sprinkle with the mint, parsley, and broken pita chips.

Toss the salad at the table and serve on individual plates.

Serves 6

PER SERVING Calories: 240; Total Fat: 17 g (3 g saturated, 10 g monounsaturated); Carbohydrates: 19 g; Protein: 5 g; Fiber: 4 g; Sodium: 588 mg

Stir-Fry Sauce with Vegetables

When it comes to stir-fry sauce, there's good, better, and best. I've found that the difference isn't always taste, but content. This stir-fry has all of the taste but none of the trials and tribulations. No MSG. No cornstarch. No refined sugar. Low sodium. A medley of flavors combines to create a soothing sauce that is right on target as a stir-fry finisher or drizzled over chicken or fish. I always keep some on hand.

INNER COOK NOTES
You can store any extra sauce in the fridge for up to 1 week or freeze for later use.

SAUCE

1 teaspoon kudzu root powder

4 tablespoons water

$1/4$ cup tamari

1 tablespoon brown rice vinegar

3 tablespoons maple syrup

$1^1/_2$ tablespoons fresh lime juice

1 teaspoon minced garlic

1 teaspoon minced fresh ginger

Pinch of cayenne

$1/4$ teaspoon toasted sesame oil

VEGETABLES

Use a variety of vegetables, for example:

2 large heads of baby bok choy, chopped, keeping leaves and stems separate

1 zucchini, thinly sliced into rounds

1 cup broccoli florets

1 carrot, thinly sliced

$1/2$ cup sliced mushrooms

1 to 2 teaspoons sesame oil

Toasted sesame seeds or cashews, for garnish (see page 151) (optional)

Judy and her daughter, Celia, are constantly looking for meals that fit Judy's comfort level. "The hardest part is incorporating vegetables in my diet. A lot of it has to do with chopping them. Too much chopping." This recipe gave them a solution. Says Celia, "Now I cut up bags of vegetables for Mom and put them in the refrigerator so she can stir-fry them." This is one recipe where others can help you out if you're too fatigued or otherwise unable to prepare vegetables.

In a small bowl, whisk the kudzu with the 2 tablespoons cold water until completely dissolved, making a slurry.

In a small saucepan over medium-high heat, combine the tamari, vinegar, 2 tablespoons water, the maple syrup, lime juice, garlic, ginger, and cayenne. Stir and bring to a boil. Decrease the heat to a simmer. The sauce will begin to thicken and reduce in volume by one-third. Stir in the slurry, whisking continuously. Mix in the sesame oil and set aside.

Cut or slice the vegetables into similar sizes for even cooking and place them in individual mounds on your cutting board. The cooking process is very fast so everything should be ready. Heat a wok or sauté pan over high heat. Add 1 or 2 teaspoons sesame oil and swirl to glaze the pan. Add your vegetables (adding the ones that take longer to cook first) and sauté for 1 to 2 minutes, depending on the veggies you choose. Add up to $1/4$ cup of the sauce mixture to coat and stir-fry for another 30 seconds, or until the vegetables are ready. Serve immediately, garnished with the sesame seeds, in a small colorful bowl.

Makes about 1 cup of sauce (Serves 4)

PER SERVING Calories: 120; Total Fat: 2 g (0 g saturated, 1 g monounsaturated); Carbohydrates: 20 g; Protein: 9 g; Fiber: 6 g; Sodium: 674 mg

String Beans with Caramelized Shallot, Rosemary, and Garlic

Learning to cook, in my mind, means being fully engaged and bringing all your senses to bear. When you learn how to do that, cooking becomes like a meditation, and it's interesting what people begin to notice. One of the class participants says that her husband claims that he can tell whether string beans are done simply by using his ears. "If you don't cook them long enough they squeak!"

I can't imagine any green bean more maligned in American culture than the string bean. The canned versions often resemble a Seattle drizzle and are about as tasty as a one-note piano (salt . . . salt . . . salt). The restaurant versions are at least pretty to look at (sometimes), but they're still bland. I'm here to tell you that string beans can have pizzazz. I start by giving them a special bath: a quick dip in boiling salted water followed by an even faster plunge into a cold pool. This parboiling cooks the beans and brings out their beautiful color.

1 teaspoon sea salt	2 tablespoons minced garlic
1 pound string beans, "tails" removed	$1/4$ teaspoon chopped fresh rosemary
2 tablespoons extra virgin olive oil	$1/4$ teaspoon grated lemon zest
2 tablespoons diced shallots	Spritz of fresh lemon juice

Fill a 4- to 6-quart pot three-fourths full with water and bring to a boil. Add the 1 teaspoon salt. Add the string beans and blanch for 3 minutes. (If you're using baby green beans, blanch for 1 minute.) Drain the string beans and place in an ice water bath. This stops the cooking process and preserves their great color.

In a sauté pan over medium heat, heat the olive oil. Add the shallots and a pinch of salt. Sauté for 3 minutes, until the shallots are golden. Add the garlic and sauté for 30 seconds more, just until aromatic.

Deglaze the pan with $1/4$ cup of water. Add the blanched string beans and a pinch of salt. Taste the beans for doneness. Add the rosemary, lemon zest, and a spritz of lemon juice. Serve immediately.

Serves 6

PER SERVING Calories: 78; Total Fat: 5 g (0 g saturated, 4 g monounsaturated); Carbohydrates: 6 g; Protein: 1 g; Fiber: 2 g; Sodium: 397 mg

Bombay Beans

The flavors of cumin and turmeric are your ticket for a virtual trip to Bombay. Another vote for "Yum!"

1¼ teaspoons sea salt

1 pound string beans, "tails" removed

2 tablespoons extra virgin olive oil

1 tablespoon diced shallot

1 teaspoon whole mustard seeds

1 teaspoon whole cumin seeds

¼ teaspoon turmeric

2 to 3 teaspoons fresh lime juice

Fill a 4- to 6-quart pot three-fourths full with water and bring to a boil. Add 1 teaspoon salt. Add the string beans and blanch for 3 minutes. (If you're using baby green beans, blanch for 1 minute.) Drain the string beans and place in an ice water bath. This stops the cooking process and preserves their great color.

In a large sauté pan over medium heat, heat the olive oil. Add the shallot, mustard seeds, and cumin seeds and sauté until golden brown (be careful: mustard seeds will pop as they heat).

Quickly add the blanched beans, ¼ teaspoon salt, and turmeric. Toss, squeeze the lime juice over the beans, and serve immediately.

Serves 6

PER SERVING Calories: 66; Total Fat: 5 g (0 g saturated, 4 g monounsaturated); Carbohydrates: 5 g; Protein: 1 g; Fiber: 2 g; Sodium: 496 mg

String Beans with Cherry Tomatoes and Feta Cheese

After parboiling the beans, it's time for a little help from some friends: a sauté of olive oil, shallots, and garlic, a sprinkle of sea salt, and a few spritzes of lemon. The result is a gorgeous green canvas on which to paint a delightful picture with tomatoes and feta cheese. While olive oil and garlic are a must for these string bean variations, for an Italian twist add caramelized shallots and rosemary.

1 teaspoon sea salt

1 pound string beans, "tails" removed

2 tablespoons extra virgin olive oil

2 shallots, diced

2 cloves garlic, chopped

$1/2$ teaspoon dried oregano

$1/4$ cup quartered cherry tomatoes

$1/3$ cup crumbled organic feta cheese

$1/4$ teaspoon chopped fresh basil, for garnish

$1/4$ teaspoon chopped fresh mint, for garnish

Fill a 4- to 6-quart pot three-fourths full with water and bring to a boil. Add the 1 teaspoon salt. Add the string beans and blanch for 3 minutes. (If you're using baby green beans, blanch for 1 minute.) Drain the string beans and place in an ice water bath. This stops the cooking process and preserves their great color.

In a sauté pan over medium heat, heat the olive oil. Add the shallots and sauté for 3 to 5 minutes, until the shallots are caramelized. Add the garlic and oregano and sauté for 30 seconds, just until aromatic.

Add the blanched beans to the sauté pan with a pinch of salt and a tablespoon of water. Reduce the heat to low and cook until tender. As they cook, taste the beans for doneness.

Put the cooked beans in a serving bowl or on a platter and toss with the tomatoes and feta. Garnish with the basil and mint and serve immediately.

Serves 6

PER SERVING Calories: 88; Total Fat: 6 g (2 g saturated, 4 g monounsaturated); Carbohydrates: 6 g; Protein: 3 g; Fiber: 2 g; Sodium: 490 mg

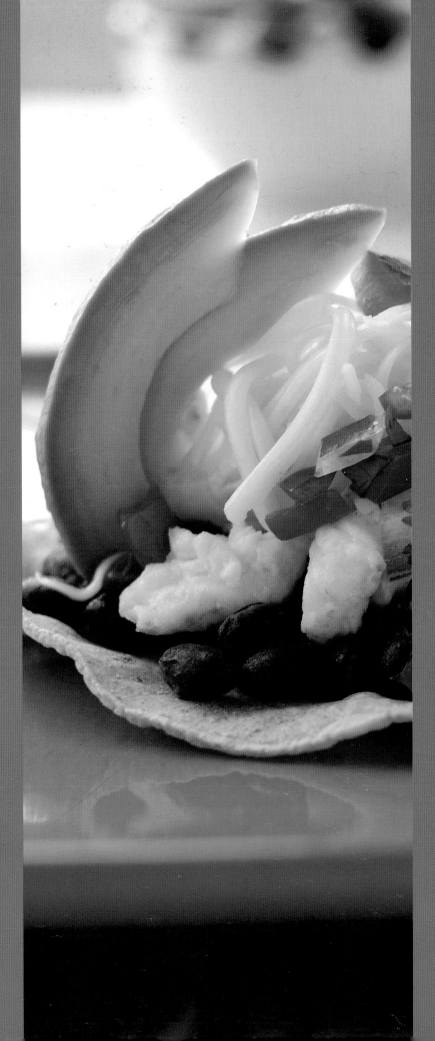

I always feel like a phys ed teacher instead of a cook when I talk about proteins. There's no way around it: The body, your body, must have proteins to survive. Proteins provide the raw materials the body requires to act like a mechanic, repairing muscles and skeletons as they break down. Everyday health depends upon getting enough protein, and this need is intensified when someone is battling cancer. I want you to get your proteins. I want you to pump yourself up.

NOW I'M PUTTING MY APRON BACK ON. There are lots of things you can eat to get protein. Nuts and eggs have protein. So do beans and grains. Each, in their own way, supplies some of the proteins we need. However, the biggest protein bang for the buck comes from fish, poultry, and meat. Without getting too scientific, people undergoing cancer treatment may need more protein than healthy persons—as much as sixty grams of protein a day during treatment, depending upon their weight. The good news is that just a 3-ounce serving of fish, poultry, or meat gets us nearly halfway there.

If you're a vegetarian, that doesn't mean you're out of luck. You can get lots of protein by drinking protein shakes, which are in the Anytime Foods chapter. However, it's not unusual for even vegetarians or very occasional meat eaters to crave animal proteins when they're sick.

If you do regularly eat fish or chicken, you might still be wondering what's the best way to eat these foods during times of illness. If you take a close look at the recipes in this section, you'll see they all have something in common: A little fish, poultry, or meat goes a long way. The dense proteins they pack are also extremely satiating, which is good news for those times when you don't feel like eating much. The truth is, when people say they want fish—or even red meat—what they're really saying is they want the taste and texture of that dish, but they

don't necessarily want a lot of it. It may come as a surprise to those of you accustomed to a humongous fillet, but that three-ounce serving can still yield the flavor and feel you crave in every bite.

Asian cuisines often use a small amount of meat in their entrées. I've had noodle dishes where the poultry is so finely sliced that I would have sworn there were six ounces of chicken in my bowl, when in reality there was far less. Using fish, poultry, or meat as part of a medley of vegetables and spices is a great way to push all your flavor buttons at once.

One last plea: Please, please, use organically grown poultry and meat. Organic poultry is not the same as "free range" products. Organic chickens and turkeys have been fed organic feed, and they haven't been shot up with antibiotics or growth hormones. All "free range" means is that your bird took a stroll someplace instead of being cooped up. Organic meat is also raised without drugs. As for fish, there are benefits to choosing those raised in clean cold-water rivers. Wild cold-water salmon, for example, have greater quantities of omega-3 fatty acids. The omega-3s have been shown to reduce inflammation; some researchers believe increased inflammation may be linked to certain cancers and cardiovascular disease. The Resource Guide in the back of the book lists sources for organic products.

Chicken Patties with Apple and Arugula

Why a pattie and not a burger? You can shape these into a poultry puck if you like, but they're ideal in bite-size proportions. They're perfect for steak-and-egg types who prefer a morning protein rush. I wouldn't recommend deep-frying because it's not necessary; grilling or pan searing is healthier and just as tasty. Apple—which is commonly added to sausage links—adds a pleasant, sweet taste that isn't overpowering. These are fast and simple to make and store well in the freezer.

2 pounds ground dark-meat organic chicken

1 cup tightly packed arugula or spinach leaves, finely chopped

1 cup peeled, diced apple

$^2/_3$ cup finely chopped onion

1 teaspoon crushed fennel seeds

$^1/_2$ teaspoon ground cumin

$^1/_2$ teaspoon sea salt

$^1/_2$ teaspoon freshly ground pepper

Spritz of fresh lemon juice

Olive oil to coat the pan or grill

In a large bowl, combine the chicken, arugula, apple, onion, fennel seeds, cumin, salt, pepper, and lemon juice and mix well. Form into desired sizes of patties.

To grill, preheat a grill pan and brush with oil. Grill the patties over medium heat until browned on both sides. Continue grilling until cooked through.

Or, in a sauté pan, add just enough oil to coat a hot pan. Sauté over medium heat for about 4 minutes on each side, until brown, then add a tablespoon of water and cover to steam until cooked through. Serve as a burger in a bun, with breakfast, or take for lunch.

Serves 8

PER SERVING Calories: 161; Total Fat: 3 g (1 g saturated, 2 g monounsaturated); Carbohydrates: 3 g; Protein: 23 g; Fiber: 0 g; Sodium: 245 mg

Chicken . . . Roasted All The Way to Yum!

Everyone I know associates a roast chicken with childhood family dinners. I used to think roasting a chicken was a huge production, probably because when I was a kid every bird seemed to be accompanied by endless side dishes. Then I went to Italy and got a crash course in roasting. I didn't have much of a choice: The signora of the house dropped a plucked duck in my lap. I barely spoke the mother-tongue, so it was pretty clear I was going to have to rely on my own wits. I got over my stage fright and figured out the tricks: a hot oven, some lemon juice, salt, and a few aromatics. It worked with the duck. It works with a chicken. And it's not a huge production.

The chicken you roast on Sunday can be used for dinner throughout the week. Instead of putting the chicken back in the refrigerator with plastic barely covering the platter, remove the meat from the bones and store in an airtight container. Save the carcass in another airtight container or bag and put it in the freezer. You can make incredible roasted chicken stock from the bones and wonderful chicken potpies from the meat.

1 (4^1/$_2$- to 5-pound) organic chicken, rinsed and thoroughly dried

1 teaspoon sea salt

1 teaspoon freshly ground pepper

2 lemons

2 sprigs fresh rosemary, or ^{1}/$_2$ teaspoon dried rosemary

2 sprigs fresh thyme, or ^{1}/$_2$ teaspoon dried thyme

2 fresh sage leaves

Preheat the oven to 450°F.

Be sure that your chicken is thoroughly dry.

Rub the chicken cavity with ^{1}/$_2$ teaspoon of the salt. Combine the remaining ^{1}/$_2$ teaspoon salt and the pepper and rub the mixture into the skin of the chicken. Cut the lemons in half and squeeze their juice over the chicken. Put the lemon rinds, rosemary, thyme, and sage into the chicken cavity.

Place the chicken on a roasting rack in a glass or ceramic dish breast side down (that's legs and butt up!).

Roast for 20 to 30 minutes, turn the chicken breast side up, and roast for another 20 to 30 minutes. Each side should be crisp and brown. You're cooking at a very high heat, so watch the timing carefully.

Decrease the heat to 350°F and continue roasting for 20 minutes, or until a meat thermometer reads 170°F when inserted in the thigh or until the juices run clear.

Serves 6

PER SERVING Calories: 264; Total Fat: 5 g (1 g saturated, 2 g monounsaturated); Carbohydrates: 0 g; Protein: 51 g; Fiber: 0 g; Sodium: 537 mg

No-Fuss Roasted Chicken Stock

Now you've had fabulous roasted chicken, but the carcass is still around. What to do?

1 carcass of a roasted organic chicken, plus any pan juices

1 medium yellow onion, with skin on, quartered

2 medium unpeeled carrots, cut into chunks

Handful of fresh flat-leaf parsley, with stems

1 stalk celery, cut into chunks

12 black peppercorns

Sachet of a sprig each of fresh rosemary and thyme with 2 fresh sage leaves (or a pinch each of dried rosemary and thyme and $1/8$ teaspoon dried sage)

$1/4$ teaspoon sea salt

Place the whole carcass in a large stockpot.

Add the onions, carrots, parsley, celery, peppercorns, herb sachet, and salt. Cover with water to 3 inches from the pot rim. Cover and bring to a boil over high heat. Uncover, decrease the heat to low, and simmer for at least an hour, until the stock has a rich flavor.

Remove from the heat and strain through a fine-mesh strainer or a colander lined with unbleached cheesecloth. (Remember that the pot is heavy and full of hot stock. Be careful!) Cool to room temperature. Store, covered, in the refrigerator for up to 1 week, or freeze for up to 3 months.

Makes about 6 quarts

PER SERVING (1 cup per serving) Calories: 75; Total Fat: 4 g (1 g saturated, 1 g monounsaturated); Carbohydrates: 1 g; Protein: 7 g; Fiber: 0 g; Sodium: 34 mg

The Big O: Imagine I'm shouting this message with a megaphone the size of the Liberty Bell, sans crack. Organic chickens are much, much, much healthier to eat! They're free of growth hormones and antibiotics that no one needs in their system. Look for a plump bird with yellowish fat instead of white and I promise you'll be able to taste the difference. Organic chickens are now so popular that you should be able to find them in your local supermarket. If not, check out the Resource Guide in the back of the book to order them online.

Lemony Chicken with Capers and Kalamata Olives

INNER COOK NOTES
Depending on the thickness of the breasts, the chicken may take a little longer to bake. Check after 15 minutes and add more liquid if the bottom of the baking dish looks dry.

For an extra dollop of yum, top with Grandma Nora's Salsa Verde (page 117).

Don't let the time needed to marinate the chicken stop you from making this recipe. Although 2 hours of marinating is my preference, even a half hour yields a succulent bird.

Here's another way to keep the bird from becoming routine. This chicken recipe is a favorite of people who don't like spending much time in the kitchen. The dish is a gentle balance of sweet and salty, as the orange juice plays well against the capers and olives. The lemon juice gives it a clean, bright Mediterranean feel. I like serving it over Garlicky Leafy Greens (see page 37).

2 boneless organic chicken breasts, halved

$1^1/_2$ teaspoons sea salt

$^1/_2$ cup fresh lemon juice

1 cup halved and thinly sliced red onion

$1^1/_2$ cups fresh orange juice

2 tablespoons extra virgin olive oil

2 teaspoons dried oregano

2 tablespoons thinly sliced garlic

2 teaspoons capers, rinsed

$^1/_4$ cup pitted kalamata olives, halved lengthwise

Preheat the oven to 375°F.

Marinate the chicken breasts with 1 teaspoon salt and $^1/_4$ cup of the lemon juice for a minimum of 30 minutes optimum and up to two hours for a spa treatment. Rinse the chicken and pat dry. Sprinkle each chicken piece with $^1/_4$ teaspoon salt.

Spread the onions in the bottom of a shallow glass baking dish. Add the orange juice and place the chicken breasts on top of the onions.

Whisk together the remaining $^1/_4$ cup lemon juice, the olive oil, and oregano. Drizzle over the chicken. Sprinkle the garlic and capers over the chicken. Add the olives to the pan juice (don't put them on top, or they will leave their mark!). Bake, uncovered, until the juices of the chicken run clear, about 30 minutes, or until an instant-read meat thermometer reads 160°F.

Transfer the chicken to a serving platter with the pan juices, olives, and capers.

Serves 4

PER SERVING Calories: 317; Total Fat: 16 g (3 g saturated, 9 g monounsaturated); Carbohydrates: 17 g; Protein: 26 g; Fiber: 1g; Sodium: 851 mg

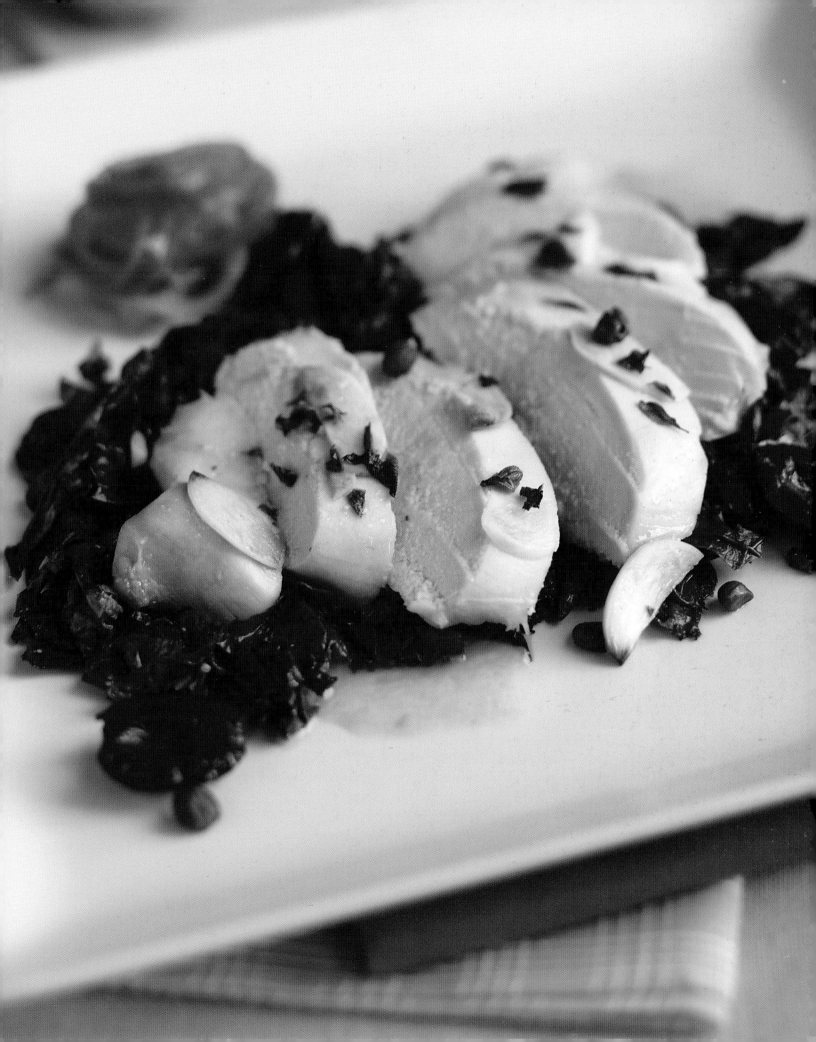

Asian Salmon Salad

This Asian salmon dish gets its flavor from ginger, lime, sesame oil, and scallions. It takes about five minutes to prepare this salad, so no more excuses that you don't have the time to make lunch!

1 (7$\frac{1}{2}$-ounce) can pink salmon

$\frac{1}{2}$ teaspoon grated fresh ginger

1 teaspoon fresh lime juice

1 tablespoon finely chopped scallions, green parts only

$\frac{1}{8}$ teaspoon sea salt

1 teaspoon sesame oil

Drain the salmon in a fine-mesh strainer and remove any bones. Place the salmon in a small bowl and use a fork to break it up. Add the ginger, lime juice, scallions, salt, and sesame oil. Mix well and taste. You may want to add a pinch of salt or a squeeze of lime.

This salmon salad would be great with Baby Bok Choy with Sesame and Ginger (page 31) or salad greens. I also love putting this salad on sesame rice crackers, dark pumpernickel, or rye.

Makes about 1 cup (Serves 4)

PER SERVING Calories: 87; Total Fat: 5 g (1 g saturated, 0 g monounsaturated); Carbohydrates: 0 g; Protein: 10 g; Fiber: 0 g; Sodium: 302 mg

Salmon Salad with Caper Salsa

I'd love to take a snapshot of someone's face when they open the pantry and come face-to-face with a can of salmon. It's the same look you see on people who have just popped the hood on their broken-down car and are staring at the engine: What the heck am I supposed to do with this? *These recipes were designed to replace that confusion with confidence. Salmon is great to eat; it's full of proteins and omega-3 fatty acids. Split a can of pink salmon in half and you can make this and the Asian Salmon Salad on page 56. This caper salsa, with red onion, olive oil, lemon juice, and dill, is reminiscent of what many people add to lox and bagels.*

1 (7^1/$_2$-ounce) can pink salmon	^{1}/$_8$ teaspoon sea salt
2 teaspoons chopped rinsed capers	^{1}/$_8$ teaspoon freshly ground pepper
2 teaspoons diced red onion	1 teaspoon extra virgin olive oil
2 teaspoons fresh lemon juice	^{1}/$_4$ teaspoon chopped fresh dill

Drain the salmon in a fine-mesh strainer and remove any bones. Place the salmon in a small bowl and use a fork to break it up. Add the capers, onion, lemon juice, salt, pepper, olive oil, and dill. Mix well and taste. You may want to add a pinch of salt, a squeeze of lemon, or a caper or two.

Serve on a bed of salad greens with water crackers or crostini. Try it as a filling for tomatoes or with scrambled eggs. Or use salmon salad instead of tuna salad for a new sandwich twist.

Serves 4

PER SERVING Calories: 88; Total Fat: 5 g (1 g saturated, 1 g monounsaturated); Carbohydrates: 0 g; Protein: 10 g; Fiber: 0 g; Sodium: 344 mg

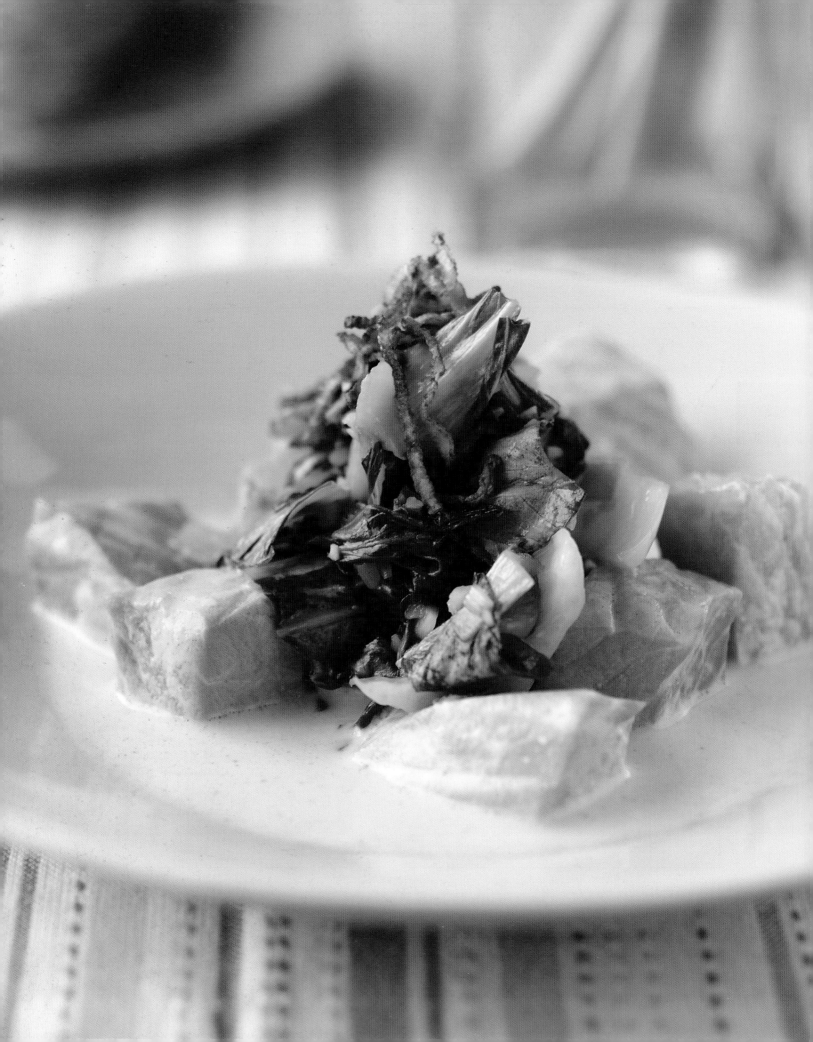

Poached Coconut Ginger Salmon

There are so many delightful flavors melded in the broth of this dish that your taste buds will be surprised and tickled. While the coconut broth puts this dish in the "cozy" food category, the infusion of ginger, lemongrass, and kaffir lime leaves adds an exotic twist. The fun part of this dish is watching the broth evolve to a pinkish hue as it cooks. That's the time to inhale deeply, taking in the aromatics. In a few minutes, you've gone from simple stock and coconut milk to a delicately balanced silky broth. That's the magic!

1 pound wild salmon fillet, pin bones removed and cut into 1-inch cubes

$^1/_2$ teaspoon sea salt

8 cups Magic Mineral Broth (page 13)

2 (14.5-ounce) cans coconut milk

3 (1-inch) pieces fresh ginger

2 shallot bulbs, halved and bruised

3 kaffir lime leaves (page 140)

1 stalk lemongrass, cut in chunks and bruised

Squeeze of fresh lime juice

Chopped scallions, fresh cilantro, or fresh mint, for garnish

Season the salmon with $^1/_4$ teaspoon salt, cover tightly, and refrigerate for a minimum of 30 minutes and up to several hours.

In a large straight-sided sauté pan or a low-sided pot just large enough to hold the salmon in a single layer, bring the broth, coconut milk, ginger, shallots, lime leaves, lemongrass, and $^1/_4$ teaspoon salt to a slow boil over medium heat. Let the ingredients infuse their flavor into the liquid for about 20 minutes. Decrease the heat to low and continue to let the broth develop for another 30 to 40 minutes; it will be worth the wait.

Remove half of the broth from the sauté pan and reserve for a future use.

Slide the salmon into the remaining broth and poach over medium heat for 7 to 9 minutes, just until tender. Serve in a shallow bowl with the broth ladled on top. Squeeze a bit of lime over each fillet and garnish with scallions, cilantro, or mint.

Serves 6

PER SERVING Calories: 413; Total Fat: 35 g (27 g saturated, 3 g monounsaturated); Carbohydrates: 8 g; Protein: 20 g; Fiber: 2 g; Sodium: 275 mg

INNER COOK NOTES

This dish is great with Baby Bok Choy with Sesame and Ginger (page 31) and Coconut Ginger Rice with Cilantro (page 100). You could even use 1 cup of the reserved broth along with water to make the rice.

Purée the reserved broth with cooked sweet potato to make a great soup such as the Sweet Potato–Coconut Soup (page 18).

This broth is no one-trick pony: it perks up chicken and vegetables as well.

Store the broth in the fridge for up to 1 week in an airtight container. Leftover cooked fish will keep in your refrigerator for 1 day and can be used in the Asian Salmon Salad (page 56).

The easiest way I know to bruise lemongrass is to cut the lemongrass into chunks with a sharp knife and use the flat side of the knife to smash each piece. This allows the full flavor of the lemongrass to be infused into the broth. Fragrant kaffir lime leaves are also referred to as wild lime leaves. If you don't have kaffir lime leaves, squeeze some fresh lime juice into the broth when it's finished.

Miso Salmon with Lime-Ginger Glaze

INNER COOK NOTES
You can grill this dish too, but use caution: the marinade can burn easily if the grill is too hot. Before grilling, wipe the marinade off the salmon, rub the salmon with a teaspoon of sesame oil, and wipe the grill with a teaspoon of sesame oil. Grill the salmon fillets over slow, even heat for about 4 minutes on each side.

This salmon is great served with Baby Bok Choy with Sesame and Ginger (page 31).

At first glance this recipe appears to be a culinary Tower of Babel: with so many flavors talking at once, you might wonder how any of them can be clearly heard. The balancing power of FASS is the reason why. Every quadrant of the taste spectrum weighs in here: the touch of sesame oil provides fat, the lime contributes the acid that unlocks the salmon's flavor, the miso gives a hint of salt, and the mirin plays the sweetheart in this fish tale. Whip up the marinade, let the salmon do the backstroke in it for a tad, and bake away. As a friend likes to say, "Tay-stee!"

3 tablespoons white miso	1 teaspoon toasted sesame oil
3 tablespoons fresh lime juice	4 (4-ounce) wild salmon fillets,
1/4 cup mirin	pin bones removed
1 tablespoon grated fresh ginger	

Whisk together the miso, lime juice, mirin, ginger, and sesame oil in a mixing bowl. Put the salmon in a baking dish, pour half the marinade over the salmon, and turn to coat well. Reserve the remaining marinade. Marinate the salmon in the refrigerator for at least 1 hour.

Preheat the oven to 400°F.

Place the salmon in a baking dish with its marinade and 1/4 cup of water. Bake for 8 to 10 minutes, or a few minutes longer if the fillets are thick.

In a saucepan, heat the reserved marinade over medium heat until it starts bubbling. When the salmon is cooked, pour the marinade over the fillets and serve immediately on a platter or individual plates.

Serves 4

PER SERVING Calories: 256; Total Fat: 9 g (1 g saturated, 3 g monounsaturated); Carbohydrates: 10 g; Protein: 27 g; Fiber: 0 g; Sodium: 409 mg

A client of mine never cooked fish until she tried this recipe. She now grills it outside in her pj's. Good thing she has a tall fence. She tells me that "my preference is for pieces of fish rather than a whole fillet, so I cut the fillet into strips. It's perfect for me." This marinade is no one-trick pony: It perks up chicken and vegetables as well. The marinade stores in the fridge for up to a week when placed in an airtight container.

Leftover cooked fish will keep in your refrigerator for 1 day and can be used in Asian Salmon Salad (page 56).

Turkey Patties

As with the chicken patties, you can go large or small. More than most meats, turkey combines well with herbs, spices, and onion. I like putting a patty on a sprouted-wheat bun with caramelized onions and slices of avocado, lettuce, and tomato. I use dark turkey meat instead of light meat because it has three times more iron per serving.

2 pounds ground dark-meat organic turkey

$^2/_3$ cup minced yellow onion

$^1/_4$ cup finely chopped fresh basil leaves

$^1/_4$ cup finely chopped fresh flat-leaf parsley

1 teaspoon minced fresh ginger

1 tablespoon minced garlic

$^1/_2$ teaspoon sea salt

1 teaspoon crushed fennel seeds

1 teaspoon dried oregano

$^1/_8$ teaspoon red pepper flakes

Olive oil for coating the pan or grill

In a large bowl, combine the turkey, onion, basil, parsley, ginger, garlic, salt, fennel, oregano, and red pepper flakes. Mix well. Shape into desired sizes of patties.

Heat a grill pan brushed with oil and brown the patties over medium heat on both sides, about 3 minutes per side. Cover and continue to grill for 3 more minutes until cooked through.

Or, in a sauté pan, add just enough oil to coat a hot pan. Sauté over medium heat for about 3 minutes on each side to brown, decrease the heat, and add a tablespoon of water. Cover to steam the inside, about 6 minutes. Serve in a pita or on a bun.

Makes 8

PER SERVING Calories: 160; Total Fat: 5 g (2 g saturated, 2 g monounsaturated); Carbohydrates: 2 g; Protein: 23 g; Fiber: 0 g; Sodium: 236 mg

Many people I work with are fast-food fans. For these people, the turkey patties at least look familiar, although they are far healthier than anything that passes through a fast-food window. One of my clients fighting cancer was a total junk fooder; when we were cleaning out his pantry he nearly cried when his wife told us to throw away his favorite fast-food coupons. He also was enamored with drive-through breakfasts. We got him to try these patties instead, topped with a little Grandma Nora's Salsa Verde (page 117). He practically broke into song. "It's like musical instruments coming together, a symphony of taste!" Musical musings aside, the important thing was that he began making and freezing the patties and started weaning himself off fast food.

Tortilla Stack with Salsa Cruda

This recipe is dedicated to Lynn, a client who loved to eat traditional huevos rancheros any time of day. With all its gooey cheese and refried beans containing lard, her favorite dish needed a culinary translation, and this is it. When you'd ask what Gary was cooking for her, she'd say, "My usual: black bean medley, salsa cruda, and organic eggs, my huevos."

This is my fun way of dressing eggs to the nines. Instead of a naked scramble, I heap them on a tortilla with some Black Bean Medley (page 85), avocado, and colorful fresh salsa cruda. Everyone asks me for breakfast ideas. This certainly fits the bill, but it also makes a great brunch. It's spectacular with a Bloody Mary, virgin or experienced.

1 (15-ounce) can black beans, drained, rinsed, and mixed with a spritz of fresh lemon or lime juice and a pinch of salt

5 tablespoons Salsa Cruda (page 121)

1/4 teaspoon ground cumin

4 small corn tortillas

4 large organic eggs

1 cup shredded organic Monterey Jack cheese (optional)

1/2 avocado, sliced, or a dollop of Avocado Cream (page 115)

In a sauté pan over medium-low heat, heat the black beans with 1 tablespoon of the salsa (more if you want some heat) and cumin.

In a dry skillet over medium-high heat, heat the tortillas one at a time, turning once, until heated through and crisp.

Prep your beans, salsa, crisped tortillas, shredded cheese, and avocado cream, then you're ready to scramble!

Break the eggs into a small mixing bowl. Add 1 tablespoon of cold water and whisk with a balloon whisk until they are foamy. Whisk at least 30 times; you will see the volume in the bowl increase as you whisk. This makes light and fluffy eggs.

Pour the egg mixture into a small nonstick skillet over medium heat. Decrease the heat to low and cook for 1 minute. Using a wooden spatula, begin to slowly move the mixture around the pan. After 2 to 3 minutes you will see the eggs begin to solidify into a perfect scramble.

For each serving, place a tortilla on a plate and top with one-fourth of the beans, eggs, cheese, avocado, and salsa. Serve with pita crisps or more tortillas.

Serves 4

PER SERVING Calories: 244; Total Fat: 9 g (2 g saturated, 4 g monounsaturated); Carbohydrates: 31 g; Protein: 12 g; Fiber: 8 g; Sodium: 422 mg

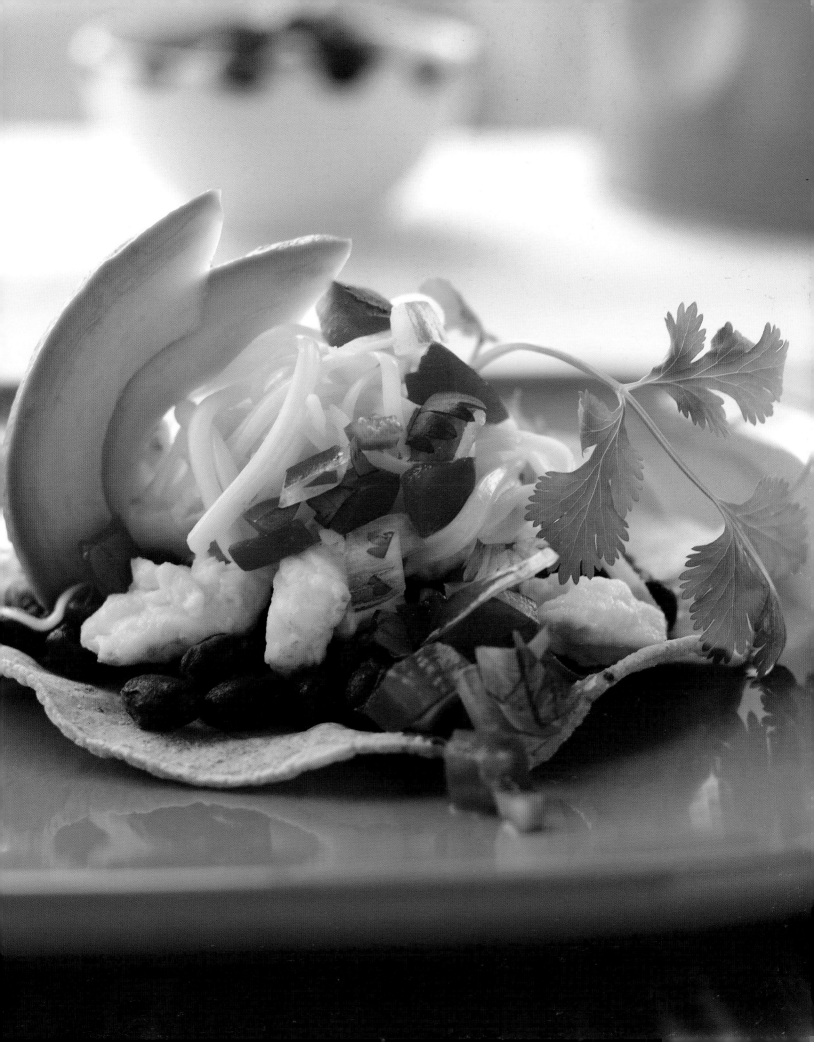

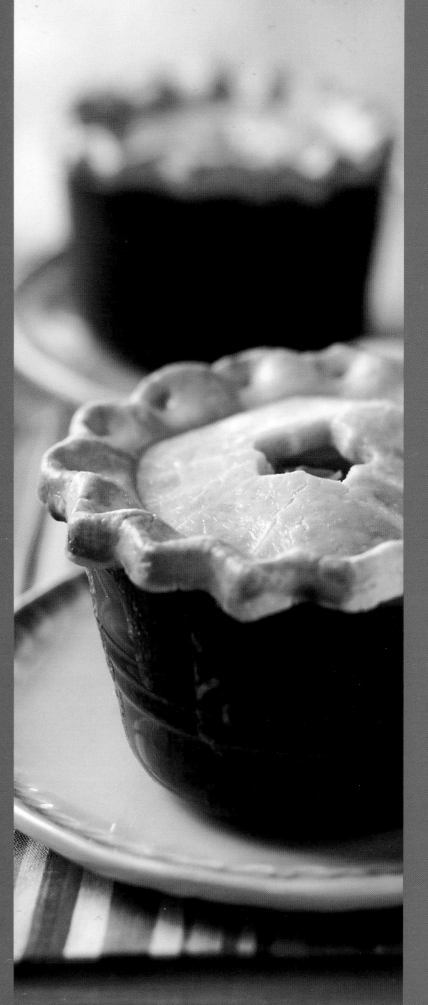

I think people underestimate their ability to take care of themselves. We tend to take for granted the everyday acts that prove my point. Cold out? Bet you're going to wear a warm coat. Need to relax? Out goes the rock and roll, in goes that ocean sounds CD. Boss not showing you the love? I see some serious comfort food in your near future.

NOW, I HAVE NOTHING AGAINST A BAG OF POTATO CHIPS OR A BIG BOWL OF ORGANIC MINT CHOCOLATE CHIP ICE CREAM. I do, however, draw the line at fast-food supersize burgers. As a friend of mine says, comfort food shouldn't leave you feeling like a beached whale.

Comfort foods have transportive qualities. They take us to a place that's safe and cozy, a space that's often reminiscent of pleasant childhood memories. Nearly everyone I know mentions some type of potatoes or pasta as their favorite comfort food. If you know a little of the science behind these foods, that makes perfect sense. Carbs in potatoes and in pasta increase our brain's serotonin levels. In turn, that elevates our mood. Carbs help put the "comfort" in comfort food.

If you're not feeling well—physically, emotionally, or otherwise—you'll find a culinary hug awaits you on every page of this chapter. That's especially important for people who are suffering from some of the side effects of cancer treatment. The recipes in this chapter are smooth and creamy. Whether it's a bowl of Creamy Polenta, or Seasonal Couscous, I guarantee each bite will go down easily and reduce your stress level. There's a combination of new and old here, with an eye toward healthy, tasty variations. If you miss macaroni and cheese but can't handle dairy, try orzo with Lemon Cashew Cream (page 119). If your tummy's a little touchy, the ginger in my mashed sweet potatoes (page 72) adds flavor while easing digestion. For traditional fare, the Chicken Potpie can't miss.

So go ahead, grab one of these friends and get comfortable. You deserve it; you've had a hard day.

Couscous Quinoa with Mint and Tomatoes

This is like pronouncing Pouilly-Fuissé; everybody messes it up. Quinoa—pronounced "keen-wah"—is an unusual grain, in both texture and nutrition; it's the only grain that is a complete protein. Here it's combined with couscous, a Mediterranean grain, and paired with fresh herbs, tomatoes, and spices.

INNER COOK NOTES
No quinoa in the house? You can make this dish entirely with couscous. Craving orange? It works well to substitute orange juice and orange zest for the lemon.

1 cup quinoa

1¼ teaspoons sea salt

1 cup couscous

2¼ teaspoons ground cumin

1⅛ teaspoons ground coriander

1 cup finely chopped fresh flat-leaf parsley

1 cup finely chopped fresh mint

2 small English cucumbers, peeled, seeded, and diced

1 cup diced tomatoes or halved cherry tomatoes

Zest of 1 lemon (about ½ teaspoon)

¼ cup fresh lemon juice

3 tablespoons extra virgin olive oil

2 scallions, green part only, finely chopped, for garnish

Place the quinoa in a fine-mesh strainer and rinse well under cold running water.

In a small saucepan, bring 1¾ cups water and 1 teaspoon salt to a boil over high heat. Add the quinoa and cover. Decrease the heat to low and simmer for 20 minutes. Remove from the heat and fluff with a fork.

While the quinoa is cooking, place the couscous in a large bowl. Add 1 cup of boiling water and ¼ teaspoon salt. Cover tightly with plastic wrap and steam for 5 minutes, or until the water is absorbed. Fluff with a fork.

Add the quinoa to the couscous, stir in the cumin and coriander, and fluff with a fork. Spread the mixture out on a sheet pan and rake with a fork occasionally until cooled.

In a large bowl, combine the parsley, mint, cucumbers, tomatoes, lemon zest and juice, and olive oil. Add the grains and mix with a fork. Chill for at least 2 hours. Now taste and think FASS: You may need a squeeze of lemon juice or a pinch of salt.

Now that you're at Yum, spoon into a large salad bowl and garnish with the scallions.

Serves 8

PER SERVING Calories: 227; Total Fat: 7 g (0 g saturated, 4 g monounsaturated); Carbohydrates: 35 g; Protein: 6 g; Fiber: 4 g; Sodium: 384 mg

Some people don't like quinoa, claiming it has a bitter taste. That's true when it's not prepared properly, as the grain is naturally coated with an off-putting resin. To get rid of the resin, put the grain in a bowl of cool water, swish it around with your hand, and drain it in a fine-mesh sieve. Repeat a bunch of times (as in five). It doesn't take that long, and it makes all the difference in this dish.

Chicken Potpie

Chicken potpie has always been my slice of scrumptious sanity. That's why it's sad to see what the frozen food folks have done with this dish. People who grew up on frozen potpies and try this recipe are astonished: The veggies aren't mealy, the crust isn't gooey, and the salt content is definitely below that of the Dead Sea. While the ingredients here are mostly traditional, I've added a few twists guaranteed to produce smiles and sighs. This is a great gift to share with someone who has a bit of the blues.

My mom, who always has an eye for color, pretties up her chicken potpies with ¹/₄ cup of green peas. Just to prove her kitchen chops, she's quick to remind me the peas are also a great source of fiber. And finally—after, what, 40 years?—she just told me her secret ingredient is a pinch of nutmeg in the sauce. It works.

2 tablespoons extra virgin olive oil

1¹/₂ cups diced yellow onion

Pinches of sea salt

³/₄ cup peeled and diced carrots

³/₄ cup diced red potato

³/₄ cup peeled and diced celery

¹/₄ teaspoon dried thyme

2 tablespoons organic unsalted butter

2 tablespoons organic unbleached all-purpose flour

¹/₂ cup All-Purpose Chicken Stock (page 9) or No-Fuss Roasted Chicken Stock (page 53)

¹/₂ cup low-fat organic milk

2 cups shredded or bite-size pieces of cooked organic chicken

Pinch of freshly ground pepper

1 recipe Potpie Pastry Crust (page 70), Tender Whole Wheat Pastry Crust (page 71), or Savory Spelt Tart Crust (page 88)

Preheat the oven to 350°F. In large sauté pan, heat the olive oil over medium heat. Add the onion and a pinch of salt. Sauté until golden. Add the carrot, potato, celery, and thyme, stir to fully incorporate, and continue to cook for 6 to 8 minutes or until just tender.

Transfer the vegetables to a bowl. In the same pan over medium-low heat, add the butter. Once it has melted, add the flour and whisk quickly to make a paste. Slowly whisk in the stock and add the milk. Keep whisking until velvety smooth. Add a pinch of salt. If the sauce is too thick, add a small amount of stock. Return the vegetables to the pan and add the chicken and a pinch of salt and pepper. Mix to combine and set aside.

Roll the prepared dough on a lightly floured surface into a circle 2 inches larger than your pie plate, and about ¹/₁₆ inch thick or roll into circles to form single serving galettes. When you make galettes be sure the mixture has cooled first. The dough for galettes is very thin and you don't want it to start cooking from the heat of the filling. Fill and bake for 20 to 30 minutes, or until the crust is golden brown. Serve hot.

Serves 6

PER SERVING Calories: 509; Total Fat: 28 g (9 g saturated, 13 g monounsaturated); Carbohydrates: 43 g; Protein: 20 g; Fiber: 7 g; Sodium: 418 mg

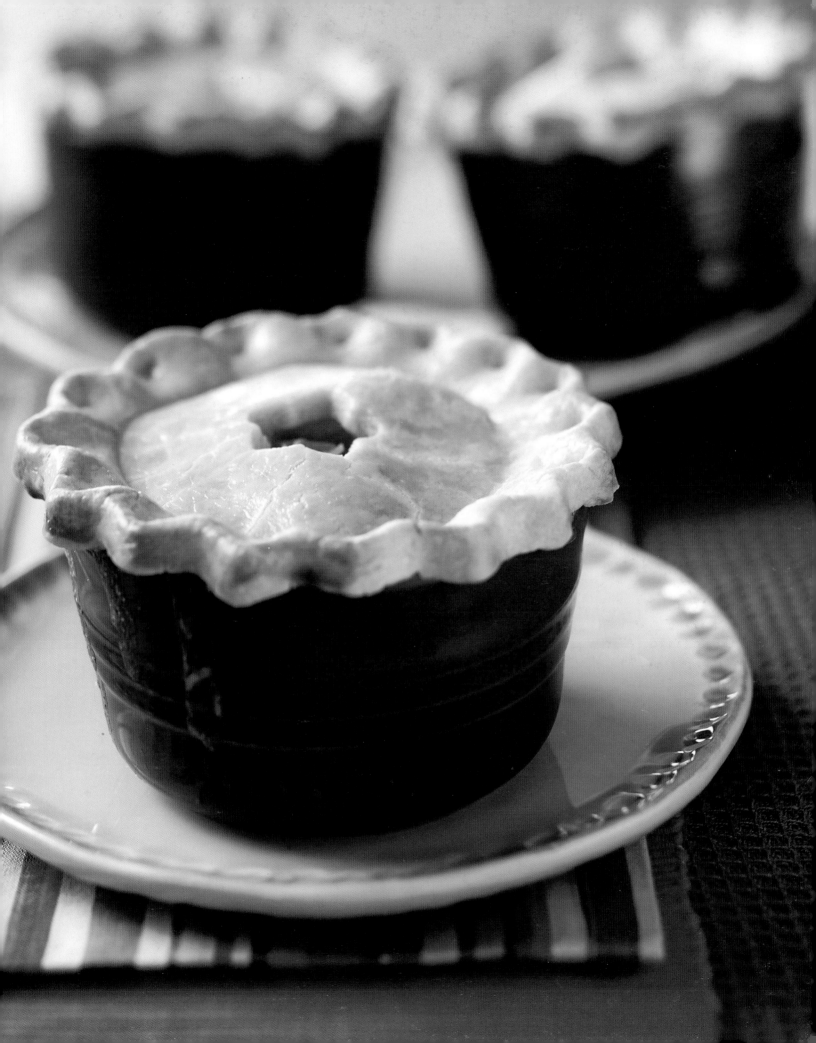

Potpie Pastry Crust

This quick and easy pastry crust uses one of my favorite culinary techniques: pressing the "go" button on my food processor. Be careful not to overprocess the pastry—you don't want it to get tough.

$^1/_2$ cup ice water

$1^1/_2$ cups organic unbleached all-purpose flour

$^3/_4$ teaspoon sea salt

6 tablespoons (3 ounces) chilled organic unsalted butter, cut into small pieces

1 organic egg, beaten in small bowl with a fork (egg wash)

In a measuring cup, add a few ice cubes to $^1/_2$ cup water. Let sit for at least 5 minutes so the water becomes very cold. Add the flour and salt to a food processor fitted with a metal blade and process for 10 seconds to combine. Add cold butter to the food processor and pulse 12 to 15 times, or until the mixture looks like coarse meal. Measure out $^1/_4$ cup ice water and pour onto flour mixture. Process for about 20 seconds, or until dough just begins to hold together. It will look very crumbly, but will hold together when pressed. Gather dough together and press into a flat disk. Wrap in plastic wrap and refrigerate for at least 30 minutes before using or freeze for up to 1 month.

Ready to roll? Scatter a bit of flour on your work surface, dust your rolling pin, and start rolling. Always roll away from yourself, turning the dough frequently as you go. Roll dough to a thickness of about $^1/_{16}$ inch.

For 4 individual ramekins: Place an empty ramekin upside down on the rolled-out dough and cut 4 circles about 1 inch larger than the ramekin. Fill the ramekins, then cut a vent in the middle of the dough circle and place on top of the filled dishes. Fold the edge over and use your fingers or a fork to press a decorative edge on the pastry. Brush the top with egg wash; bake as directed.

For 1 large pie: Place an empty pie plate upside down on the rolled dough and cut a circle about 1 inch larger than the plate. Fill plate with pie filling. Place dough on top of the filled pie plate. Fold edges over and crimp with your fingers or a fork. Cut vents into the top using a paring knife. Brush with egg wash and bake as directed.

Serves 6

PER SERVING Calories: 212; Total Fat: 12 g (7 g saturated, 3 g monounsaturated); Carbohydrates: 22 g; Protein: 4 g; Fiber: 1 g; Sodium: 308 mg

---

INNER COOK NOTES

For the most beautiful top crust, make your pastry in advance. The trick here is simply to chill the pastry for at least one hour in the refrigerator before rolling. After rolling out your pastry, cut the tops and place them on a baking sheet covered with wax paper. Chill for at least 30 minutes. Cut the center vent with a paring knife, fold the edges in, and crimp decoratively. Chill again for 30 minutes before placing on top of the cooled pie filling. Brush with an egg wash and bake as directed.

The daughter of a friend of mine, fourteen, was given a homework assignment by her teacher: Make a chicken potpie with your family and write a report. The class was told to go to a store and buy canned chicken, canned peas, canned soup, and frozen pie dough. The daughter, who had been raised on fresh foods, took one look at the list of ingredients and said to herself, "No way. I'm doing this right." Her brother got a video recorder and taped the family making this pie from scratch. The teacher took one look at the tape and her paper—they also brought her a small potpie to sample—and gave the girl an A. That kid has a place in my kitchen whenever she's ready.

Tender Whole Wheat Pastry Crust

Here's a twist on traditional white flour pastry crust that uses healthier whole wheat pastry flour instead. You won't be dissapointed.

2 cups whole wheat pastry flour

$^1/_2$ teaspoon sea salt

4 tablespoons ($^1/_2$ stick) cold organic unsalted butter, cut into small cubes

$^1/_4$ cup extra virgin olive oil

1 teaspoon maple syrup

$^1/_4$ to $^1/_3$ cup ice water

1 organic egg, beaten in small bowl with a fork (egg wash)

Add the flour and salt to a food processor fitted with a metal blade and process for 10 seconds. Remove lid and add butter and olive oil; pulse about 10 times or until a coarse meal forms. Stir the maple syrup into $^1/_4$ cup of the ice water. Pour water into the processor and pulse until coarsely mixed. The dough should hold together when pinched. If it is too dry, sprinkle in another tablespoon of the ice water and pulse a few more times to mix. Gather the dough together into a ball and press into a flat disk; wrap in plastic wrap and refrigerate for at least one hour. At this point the dough can be rolled out or wrapped in foil and stored in the freezer for up to 1 month.

Scatter a bit of pastry flour on your work surface, dust the top of the dough, and start rolling. Always roll away from yourself, turning the dough frequently as you go. Dust lightly with flour only as needed to prevent sticking. Roll dough to a thickness of about $^1/_{16}$ inch and about 2 inches larger than your pie plate. Cut the center vent before transferring the dough to the dish. Gently place the dough over the filled pie dish, brush with egg wash, and bake as directed. If you are rolling out your pastry in advance, transfer to a sheet of wax paper on a cookie sheet.

Serves 6

PER SERVING Calories: 296; Total Fat: 17 g (6 g saturated, 8 g monounsaturated); Carbohydrates: 31 g; Protein: 4 g; Fiber: 5 g; Sodium: 251 mg

INNER COOK NOTES
You can cut the vent and brush your pastry crust with the egg wash ahead of time, then place in the refrigerator until ready to use.

My dear friend Wendy Remer, baker and chocolatier extraordinaire, wanted me to give you a gentle reminder: Only use whole wheat pastry flour! Do not substitute whole wheat flour in this recipe—whole wheat pastry flour is milled much finer than regular whole wheat flour and therefore makes a tender crust instead of the sometimes tough, cardboard-tasting crust made from regular whole wheat flour. Whole wheat pastry flour is readily available in bulk, on the shelves at your local market, and by mail order from King Arthur Flour or Bob's Red Mill to name a few.

Mashed Ginger Sweet Potatoes with Fresh Nutmeg

Can I hear a "hallelujah!" for the healing power of the mighty spud? Yes, brothers and sisters, whether you are followers of the lumpy or smooth denomination, to be human is to believe in all things mashed. From Yukon to yam, the pulverized potato provides unparalleled comfort. Many of my clients going through chemotherapy swear by sweet potatoes. The ginger and nutmeg give these spuds a little moxie and help them go down quietly.

4 cups peeled and cubed sweet potatoes or yams (about 2-inch cubes)

1 teaspoon sea salt

2 tablespoons organic unsalted butter

$^1/_2$ teaspoon grated fresh ginger

$^1/_4$ teaspoon maple syrup

Pinch of ground cinnamon

Pinch of freshly grated nutmeg

Bring a large pot of water to a boil over high heat. Add the sweet potatoes and salt and cook until tender, about 25 minutes. Drain, reserving $^1/_4$ cup of the cooking liquid, and return the sweet potatoes to the pot. Add the butter, ginger, maple syrup, cinnamon, nutmeg, and 2 to 3 tablespoons of the reserved cooking liquid. Use a potato masher or electric hand mixer to mash the potatoes. Taste; you may want to add a pinch or two of salt. Serve immediately in a bowl or as a side dish on a plate.

Serves 6

PER SERVING Calories: 110; Total Fat: 4 g (2 g saturated, 1 g monounsaturated); Carbohydrates: 18 g; Protein: 1 g; Fiber: 3 g; Sodium: 442 mg

Mashed Yukon Gold Potatoes with Rutabaga

High in antioxidant properties and with a mild sweet flavor, rutabaga cohabits agreeably with potato, especially when a little nutmeg is thrown into the mix. I grew up on this dish, though if I'd known as a kid that it was so healthy, I probably wouldn't have eaten it.

2 cups peeled and cubed rutabaga (about 1-inch cubes)

1 teaspoon sea salt

2 pounds peeled and cubed Yukon gold potatoes (about 1-inch cubes)

2 tablespoons organic unsalted butter

2 to 3 tablespoons organic low-fat milk

$1/4$ teaspoon freshly grated nutmeg

Bring a large pot of water to a boil over high heat. Add the rutabaga and salt, lower the heat slightly, and boil for 10 minutes. Add the potatoes and boil until both are tender, another 15 minutes. Drain in a colander and return to the pot over low heat. Add the butter and milk. Using a potato masher or electric hand mixer, mash to the desired consistency. Add the nutmeg and taste the potatoes; you may need a pinch or two of salt or another pinch of nutmeg. Serve immediately in a colorful bowl.

Serves 6

PER SERVING Calories: 175; Total Fat: 4 g (2 g saturated, 1 g monounsaturated); Carbohydrates: 32 g; Protein: 3 g; Fiber: 4 g; Sodium: 412 mg

INNER COOK NOTES
The milk can be replaced with stock or reserved cooking liquid.

For a variation on this dish, substitute 2 cups peeled and cubed celeriac for the rutabaga and proceed as directed. Celeriac, or celery root, provides a nice, mellow taste while tempering the starchiness of the spuds. Add $1/4$ teaspoon horseradish or wasabi—or both—for some heat.

Pantry Pasta

I learned to make pasta the genuine Italian way, by having it hurled out a window by a bona fide signora *yelling that it was 40 seconds past al dente. In an operatic sort of way I learned an important lesson: Never walk away from the pasta pot. The* signora *also insisted I salt the water after it boils. Why? Who knows? I wasn't about to argue with the* signora *and risk flying out the window myself. I've since learned that pasta is an ideal canvas to feature vegetables. Serve pasta as a main course or a side dish. Either way, follow the pasta prep directions below. Otherwise the* signora *might show up at your door.*

1 teaspoon sea salt

1 pound whole wheat or spelt penne pasta

2 tablespoons extra virgin olive oil

2 tablespoons finely chopped shallot

2 teaspoons finely chopped garlic

Pinch of red pepper flakes

$^1/_4$ cup Pistachio Mint Pesto (page 25) or Basil and Arugula Pesto (page 115)

1 (15-ounce) can cannellini or white navy beans, drained, rinsed, and mixed with a spritz of fresh lemon juice and a pinch of sea salt

$^1/_4$ cup kalamata olives, pitted and halved lengthwise

1 cup sliced artichokes (canned or jarred in water, rinsed and mixed with a spritz of lemon juice and a pinch of sea salt)

Pinch of freshly grated nutmeg

$^1/_8$ to $^1/_4$ cup freshly grated organic Parmesan cheese (optional)

Bring 4 quarts of water to a boil over high heat. Add the salt. Add the pasta and cook until al dente; remember to taste at 6 minutes. When the pasta is al dente, drain, reserving $^1/_2$ cup of the cooking liquid. Set both aside.

While the pasta is cooking, heat the olive oil in a large sauté pan over medium heat. Add the shallot and sauté for 3 minutes. Add the garlic and red pepper flakes and sauté for 30 seconds, just until aromatic. Deglaze with $^1/_4$ cup of the reserved pasta cooking liquid. Add the hot cooked pasta and the pesto to the pan.

Add the beans, olives, artichokes, and the remaining $^1/_4$ cup of the reserved cooking liquid. Stir until well combined and creamy. Stir in the nutmeg and cheese and serve immediately in a large bowl to bring to the table or individual pasta bowls.

Serves 6

PER SERVING Calories: 434; Total Fat: 10 g (1 g saturated, 5 g monounsaturated); Carbohydrates: 71 g; Protein: 14 g; Fiber: 10 g; Sodium: 815 mg

Swiss Chard Pasta

After the signora *threw my pasta out the window, she taught me how to make this simple dish. Pasta is a great vehicle for showcasing the versatility and tastiness of dark leafy greens. The subtle and creamy sauce is created by using the pasta water in combination with the olive oil and cheese.*

2 bunches Swiss chard, stemmed and cut into small bite-size pieces

1 teaspoon sea salt

1 pound whole wheat or spelt penne pasta

2 tablespoons extra virgin olive oil

1 tablespoon finely chopped garlic

$^1/_8$ teaspoon red pepper flakes

$^1/_4$ cup freshly grated organic Parmesan cheese (optional)

$^1/_4$ teaspoon freshly grated nutmeg

Spritz of fresh lemon juice

$^1/_4$ cup toasted walnuts, pine nuts, or pistachios (see page 151)

(see page 151)

> **INNER COOK NOTES**
> If you're not using the cheese, add only $^1/_4$ cup of the reserved cooking liquid.
>
> Substitute spinach or other greens for the Swiss chard. Or add $^1/_2$ cup halved cherry tomatoes or 1 roasted and cubed delicata squash just before adding the cheese.

Cover the chard with a cold water bath and set aside.

Bring 4 quarts of water to a boil over high heat. Add 1 teaspoon salt. Add the pasta and cook for 6 to 8 minutes (spelt or whole wheat pasta may take a little longer, but don't walk away—it doesn't take that long). Taste after 6 minutes; the pasta should still be al dente. Drain the pasta, reserving $^1/_2$ cup of the cooking liquid. Set both aside.

While the pasta is cooking, heat the olive oil in a large sauté pan over medium heat. Add the garlic and red pepper flakes and sauté for 30 seconds, just until aromatic. Lift the greens out of their cold water bath and add them, along with a bit of salt, to the sauté pan. Sauté for about 4 minutes, until tender (the water that adheres to the wet greens should be enough liquid to wilt them during cooking).

Add the pasta and $^1/_4$ cup of the reserved cooking liquid. Stir to combine. Add the cheese, nutmeg, and lemon juice. Taste: You may need some of the remaining reserved pasta water, another spritz of lemon juice, or a generous pinch of salt.

Stir in the nuts and serve immediately.

Serves 6

PER SERVING Calories: 370; Total Fat: 10 g (1 g saturated, 4 g monounsaturated); Carbohydrates: 59 g; Protein: 11 g; Fiber: 8 g; Sodium: 483 mg

Seasonal Couscous

Couscous is a southern Mediterranean staple made out of durum wheat and resembles grains. Israeli couscous is a little fatter, more like a pearl, but is still small enough to eat with a spoon. Like pasta, couscous goes great with seasonal veggies.

SQUASH

1/4 teaspoon ground cumin

1/4 teaspoon ground coriander

1/4 teaspoon sea salt

1/8 teaspoon ground cinnamon

2 tablespoons extra virgin olive oil

2 cups peeled and diced acorn squash, butternut squash, sweet potato, or a combination

COUSCOUS

1 cup couscous

1 tablespoon extra virgin olive oil

1 tablespoon diced shallot

3 tablespoons diced fennel

1/2 cup dried cranberries or currants, or a combination

Pinch of red pepper flakes

1/4 teaspoon ground cumin

1/4 teaspoon ground coriander

1/4 teaspoon sea salt

To make the squash, preheat the oven to 350°F.

In a large bowl, mix the cumin, coriander, salt, cinnamon, and olive oil. Toss the diced squash in the mixture to coat well. Roast on a rimmed sheet pan for 15 minutes, or until just tender, shaking the pan once so the squash cooks evenly. Remove from the oven, let cool, and set aside.

To make the couscous, combine the couscous and 1 cup boiling water in a large bowl and immediately cover tightly with plastic wrap. Let sit for 10 to 15 minutes, or until the moisture is absorbed. Place the couscous on a sheet pan and spread it out with a fork, raking several times while cooling to keep the grains from clumping.

While the couscous is cooling, heat the olive oil in a large sauté pan. Add the shallot and fennel and cook until soft. Add the dried cranberries, red pepper flakes, cumin, coriander, and salt. Stir well.

When the couscous has cooled, add the shallot mixture and squash. Stir well and taste; you may want a squeeze of lemon juice.

Serve at room temperature.

Serves 6

PER SERVING Calories: 220; Total Fat: 7 g (1 g saturated, 5 g monounsaturated); Carbohydrates: 35 g; Protein: 4 g; Fiber: 3 g; Sodium: 202 mg

Veggie "Ricotta" Lasagna

Talk about a recipe: When my mother first coaxed this gem out of her Italian cousin Marjorie, the notes took up four recipe cards (front and back). It also took two days to make. Sure it tasted great, but we were all exhausted from the effort. So I tinkered a little. I won't kid you: lasagna is never a meal that can be whipped up in 15 minutes, but this version of Marjorie's lasagna only takes an hour. It's worth the effort, especially because lasagna is a dish best made (and shared) by more than one pair of hands.

1 recipe Herbed "Ricotta" (page 118) or organic ricotta cheese (15 ounces)

6 cups Garlicky Leafy Greens (page 37), excess liquid squeezed out

10 ounces lasagna noodles (or Vita Spelt lasagna noodles)

4 red onions

2 tablespoons extra virgin olive oil

Pinch of sea salt

3 cups roasted tomatoes (see page 120) or 1 (16-ounce) jar of Muir Glen chunky-style prepared sauce

$1/4$ cup freshly grated organic Parmesan cheese

Preheat the oven to 350°F. Lightly coat an 8 by 10-inch or a 9 by 9-inch baking dish with olive oil.

Prepare the "ricotta," the greens, and the lasagna noodles (per package instructions) so they are ready for assembly.

Quarter the onions and thinly slice. In a large sauté pan, heat the olive oil over medium heat. Add the onions and salt. Sauté over medium heat, decrease the heat to low, and simmer for 20 minutes, until caramelized.

To assemble the lasagna, ladle $1/2$ cup of the tomato sauce into the bottom of the prepared baking dish. Place in a layer of noodles, slightly overlapped, and top with a layer of "ricotta." Spread one-third of the greens on top, top with one-third of the onions, and add another $1/2$ cup tomato sauce to the dish. Repeat until all the ingredients are used.

Sprinkle the Parmesan cheese on top. Bake, covered, for 30 minutes. Uncover and bake for 15 minutes more, or until the top is browned and bubbly. Remove from the oven and let set for 15 minutes before cutting into serving-size squares.

Serves 8

PER SERVING Calories: 462; Total Fat: 22 g (4 g saturated, 11 g monounsaturated); Carbohydrates: 53 g; Protein: 19 g; Fiber: 7 g; Sodium: 600 mg

There's something about lasagna that brings people comfort during chaos. As one client's daughter said, "I routinely made this for my mom during her treatment. It was a dish we could always count on."

We all know that half the fun of making a big lasagna is being able to serve the leftovers again and again. I suggest serving half the lasagna. Cut the rest into squares and wrap and freeze each square individually. Reheat for a quick meal.

Spinach Orzo with Pine Nuts and Feta

The Big O: I've heard farmers call spinach a "heavy feeder." That's because it pulls lots of nutrients from the soil to help it grow quickly. Spinach will gobble up everything in its path, meaning more minerals if the soil is pesticide free, and a whole bunch of nasty stuff if it's not, including fungicides and other chemicals that zap out nutrients and taste. Use organic spinach to get the most nutritional benefits.

Orzo is pasta that looks and acts like rice. Orzo is more forgiving than pasta if it's left on the stove top a tad too long. This recipe is great when served warm or at room temperature. It also works well as a pasta salad.

1 tablespoon extra virgin olive oil

$^1/_2$ cup finely chopped red onion

1 teaspoon finely chopped garlic

1 pound fresh spinach, finely chopped (about 2 cups)

$^1/_4$ cup crumbled organic feta cheese

1 teaspoon fresh lemon juice

1 tablespoon grated lemon zest

Freshly grated nutmeg

Pinch of ground cinnamon

$^1/_2$ teaspoon sea salt

1 cup orzo

$^1/_4$ cup chopped toasted pine nuts, walnuts, or pistachios (page 151), plus extra for garnish

In a large sauté pan, heat the olive oil over medium heat. Add the onion and a pinch of salt and sauté until golden. Add the garlic and sauté for 30 seconds, just until aromatic. Add the spinach and a pinch of salt and cook until wilted and tender. Add the cheese, lemon juice and zest, nutmeg, and cinnamon. Mix thoroughly.

Bring 2 quarts of water to a boil in a covered pot over high heat. Add $^1/_2$ teaspoon salt and the orzo. Cook for 8 to 10 minutes, until al dente. Drain the orzo and transfer to a large bowl. Add the spinach mixture and the $^1/_4$ cup nuts and combine.

Taste, adding a pinch of salt or another shave of nutmeg if necessary. Serve in a bowl or on a plate topped with some additional nuts.

Serves 6

PER SERVING Calories: 195; Total Fat: 7 g (1 g saturated, 2 g monounsaturated); Carbohydrates: 26 g; Protein: 8 g; Fiber: 7 g; Sodium: 328 mg

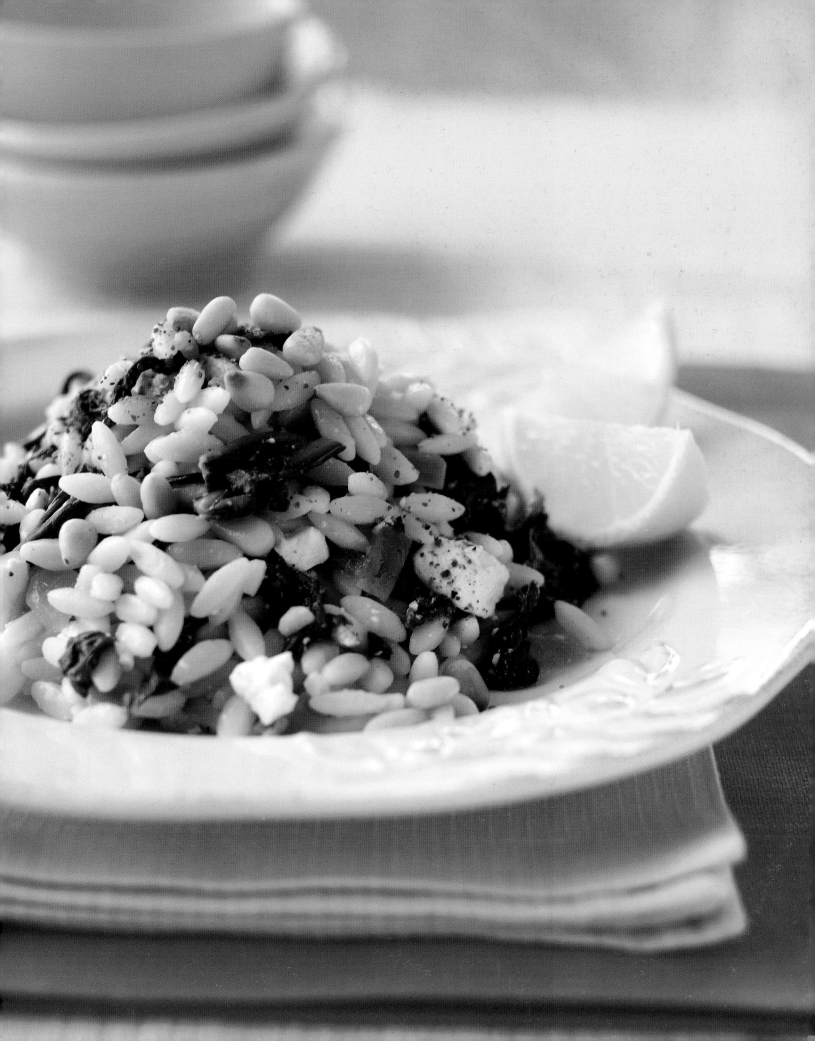

Creamy Polenta and Stacked Polenta Pie with Garlicky Greens and Puttanesca Sauce

When people ask what polenta is, I answer, "It's Italian for grits!" Polenta is ground cornmeal and a staple of northern Italian fare. Like American grits, polenta provides a foundation for many flavors. It's easy to work with, eat, and get filled up on. It's low-fat, too. The polenta pie allows greens to go undercover, especially with the Puttanesca Sauce on top. See the sidebar for a variation—the polenta bites are personal nibbles with a confetti of vegetables.

CREAMY POLENTA

1/2 teaspoon sea salt

Spritz of fresh lemon juice

1 cup polenta

2 tablespoons extra virgin olive oil

1/4 cup freshly grated organic Parmesan cheese (optional)

1 recipe Garlicky Leafy Greens (page 37)

1 recipe Puttanesca Sauce (page 120)

To make the creamy polenta, bring 4 cups of water to a boil over high heat. Add the salt and lemon juice. Very slowly add the polenta in a steady stream, whisking constantly with a wire whisk. Immediately decrease the heat to low. Continue to stir with a wooden spoon until smooth. Add the olive oil and stir the mixture constantly for about 15 minutes. Stir in the cheese.

To make stacked polenta pie, preheat the oven to 350°F. Lightly oil an 8-inch glass pie pan. Pour half the creamy polenta into the prepared pan and quickly spread evenly. Spread the greens in an even layer over the polenta. Spread the second half of the polenta over the greens, top with a sprinkle of cheese, and bake for about 10 minutes, or until the cheese is golden.

Remove from the oven and cool for about 5 minutes before cutting into wedges. To serve, place a wedge on a plate and top with Puttanesca Sauce.

Makes one 8-inch pie (Serves 6)

PER SERVING Calories: 313; Total Fat: 16 g (2 g saturated, 9 g monounsaturated); Carbohydrates: 35 g; Protein: 7 g; Fiber: 5 g; Sodium: 827 mg

---

INNER COOK NOTES

For easy polenta clean up, use cold water to clean the pan, as warm or hot water makes a sticky mush!

To make 24 mini polenta muffins, preheat the oven to 425°F and oil a mini muffin tin or fill it with paper liners. Make the Creamy Polenta using 1 cup less water and half the salt. Add 1 1/2 cups very finely diced vegetables (such as a combination of red bell pepper, zucchini, and carrot) and 1/4 cup Parmesan cheese. Stir to combine. Quickly spoon the mixture into the muffin tin and cool to room temperature, about 30 minutes. Release the polenta bites by turning the tin over and tapping the bottom, or gently release each by running a fork around the edge. Allow the bites to dry on a cooling rack for 45 minutes to an hour. Transfer (right side up) to a cookie sheet and crisp in the oven for 3 to 5 minutes. Top with your favorite pesto.

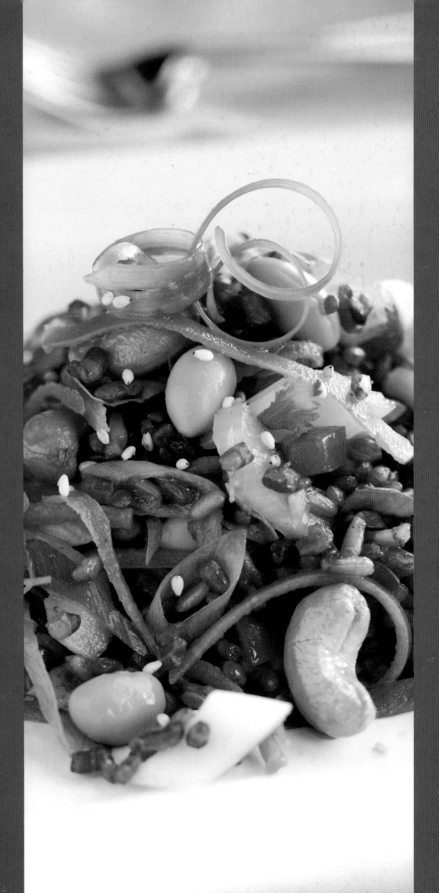

Chapter 6 Anytime Foods

I mentioned in the introduction to this book the importance of being a "flexitarian." That applies to both what you eat and when you eat it. In other words, eat when you feel hungry. If that's on a "normal" schedule—breakfast at seven, lunch at noon, dinner at six—great. But many people undergoing treatment may have cravings at odd hours, and they feel like having only a nibble rather than a feast. It's for these folks—and for people on the go—that we've come up with these portable, nutrient-packed, yummy morsels.

NOW YOU MIGHT SEE THESE RECIPES AS SNACKS, AND THAT'S FINE. I see them as something more, something akin to little appetite life rafts. Most of us view a snack as something to tide us over until we have a bigger meal. Cancer patients may go through weeks when they don't want that bigger meal because their appetites are depressed. It's at these times that they can completely lose their connection to food and drop weight rapidly. These snacks can keep their appetites afloat until their desire to eat rebounds (as it often does during a treatment cycle). That's why it's important to pack a lot of taste and health into every bite—because a few bites (or sips, in the case of the smoothies) may be all someone is able to eat.

We've mixed it up here to keep those taste buds engaged. The Pecans Spiced with Orange Zest and Ginger (page 95) and Spiced Roasted Almonds (page 99) make great highway and office nibbles. At home, a shot of smoothie (yes, I serve them that way) is a quick pick-me-up. And I promise that the Anytime Crunch (opposite) blows away those sugar-laden commercial granola bars.

So snack away all day, if you like. It's okay. In fact, I insist.

Anytime Crunch

Some words transport us right back to childhood: double-Dutch, recess, and for me, gorp. This was a special food mix I used to get when I was a young camper just before climbing a mountain. (OK, so maybe it was a hill; when you're young, hills tend to look like Everest.) Gorp was a combo of pure energy foods: peanuts, M&M's, raisins, and Chex Mix. It must have done something, because I used to run up those mountains on a sugar-high worthy of a ride on the Coney Island Cyclone. Here's a healthier version of a crunchy, satisfying energy snack for us on-the-go types. This combination of cashews and almonds mixed with the warming spices of cinnamon, cardamom, and orange zest is a nice alternative to heavily refined sugar-laden snacks found on supermarket shelves.

¹/₃ cup maple syrup

1 tablespoon extra virgin olive oil

¹/₂ teaspoon vanilla extract

³/₄ teaspoon pumpkin pie spice (or ¹/₄ teaspoon each of ground ginger, ground cinnamon and freshly grated nutmeg)

¹/₈ teaspoon sea salt

2 teaspoons grated orange zest

1 cup rolled oats

1 cup raw almonds, coarsely chopped

1 cup raw walnuts, coarsely chopped

¹/₂ cup shredded unsweetened coconut

2 tablespoons sesame seeds

Preheat the oven to 350°F. Have a baking sheet covered with parchment paper ready.

In a small bowl, whisk together the maple syrup, oil, vanilla, spices, salt, and orange zest. In a large bowl, combine the oats, almonds, walnuts, coconut, and sesame seeds. Mix well. Pour the liquid mixture over the dry ingredients and stir until well coated.

Scrape the mixture onto the baking sheet covered with parchment paper. Flatten and spread the mixture on the pan so that the grains and nuts brown evenly. Bake for 10 minutes. Remove the pan from the oven and carefully stir the grains, then spread and flatten them again. Return the pan to the oven and bake for 8 to 10 minutes longer, or until golden brown. Cool completely on the baking sheet and then transfer them to an airtight container; store for up to 1 week.

Makes about 3 cups

PER SERVING Calories: 168; Total Fat: 12 g (2 g saturated, 4 g monounsaturated); Carbohydrates: 11 g; Protein: 4 g; Fiber: 2 g; Sodium: 22 mg

Best Oatmeal Ever

Wow, do we ever mangle oatmeal in this country! Oatmeal is so easy to overcook or undercook that it usually comes out somewhere between sawdust and wall spackle. Most people lay on the butter and brown sugar to cover up these abominations. The result is a bowlful of flavored yuck. That's a shame, because when done properly, oatmeal serves as an excellent nutritional base for a heartwarming meal. So how do we get to the Best Oatmeal Ever? Part of the secret is in preparation, getting the oats to the right consistency. Keep reading to see how we pull that off. Then apply the right combination of flavors. This oatmeal has warming spices, and dried fruit also goes into the mix. Top the whole thing off with nuts or fruit compote and you'll never look at oatmeal as spackle again!

1 cup rolled or steel-cut oats

$1^1/_2$ tablespoons fresh lemon juice

$^1/_8$ teaspoon sea salt

$^1/_4$ cup dried cranberries, cherries, raisins, currants, or a mixture

$^1/_4$ teaspoon ground cinnamon

$^1/_8$ teaspoon ground cardamom

$^1/_8$ teaspoon powdered ginger or grated fresh ginger

1 teaspoon maple syrup

$^1/_4$ cup organic milk or soy milk (optional)

Chopped toasted almonds or walnuts (see page 151), or a dollop of Fruit Compote (page 116), for garnish

Place the oats in a pan or bowl with water to cover and add the lemon juice. Soak over-night. Drain through a fine-mesh sieve and rinse well under cold water.

In a 4-quart pot, combine the oats, 2 cups water, and the salt. Bring to a boil over high heat and cover. Decrease the heat to a simmer and cook for 10 minutes, stirring occasionally. Add the dried fruit, cinnamon, cardamom, and ginger. The oatmeal will become very creamy as the water evaporates. Add the maple syrup and milk and stir. For less-moist oatmeal, leave the lid off for the last 3 to 4 minutes of cooking.

Serve in a colorful bowl; garnish with toasted nuts or a dollop of compote.

Serves 2

PER SERVING Calories: 219; Total Fat: 2 g (0 g saturated, 0 g monounsaturated); Carbohydrates: 42 g; Protein: 7 g; Fiber: 5 g; Sodium: 148 mg

Black Bean Medley for Wraps with Avocado Cream

This dish looks like confetti and acts like its many colors . . . versatile! The medley—which includes red bell peppers, cumin, cinnamon, and cilantro—makes a great filling for burritos. It's also delightful over scrambled eggs with a little salsa cruda.

1 (15-ounce) can organic black beans, drained, rinsed, and mixed with a pinch of salt and a squeeze of lemon, or 2 cups cooked from dried black beans (page 150)

$^1/_4$ cup finely chopped red bell pepper

$^1/_4$ teaspoon seeded, ribbed, and finely chopped jalapeño pepper

3 tablespoons extra virgin olive oil

1 tablespoon fresh lime juice

$^1/_4$ teaspoon maple syrup

$^1/_4$ teaspoon sea salt

3 tablespoons chopped scallions, white and green parts

3 tablespoons finely chopped fresh cilantro

$^1/_4$ teaspoon ground cumin

$^1/_8$ teaspoon ground cinnamon

$^1/_2$ cup Avocado Cream (page 115), for garnish

$^1/_2$ cup Salsa Cruda (page 121), for garnish

In a medium bowl, mix the black beans, bell pepper, jalapeño, olive oil, lime juice, maple syrup, salt, scallions, cilantro, cumin, and cinnamon. Taste; you may need a pinch or two of salt or a spritz of lime juice. Spoon into a bowl and garnish with the avocado cream and/or salsa.

Makes about 2$^1/_2$ cups (Serves 6)

PER SERVING Calories: 129; Total Fat: 7 g (1 g saturated, 5 g monounsaturated); Carbohydrates: 19 g; Protein: 4 g; Fiber: 5 g; Sodium: 353 mg

INNER COOK NOTES

Heat a flour tortilla in a dry, hot pan, for about 30 seconds on each side. Remove from the heat and add the Black Bean Medley and $^1/_4$ cup cooked brown rice. Roll up the tortilla and top with Avocado Cream and/or Salsa Cruda. Also try this Black Bean Medley in the Tortilla Stack with Salsa Cruda (page 62).

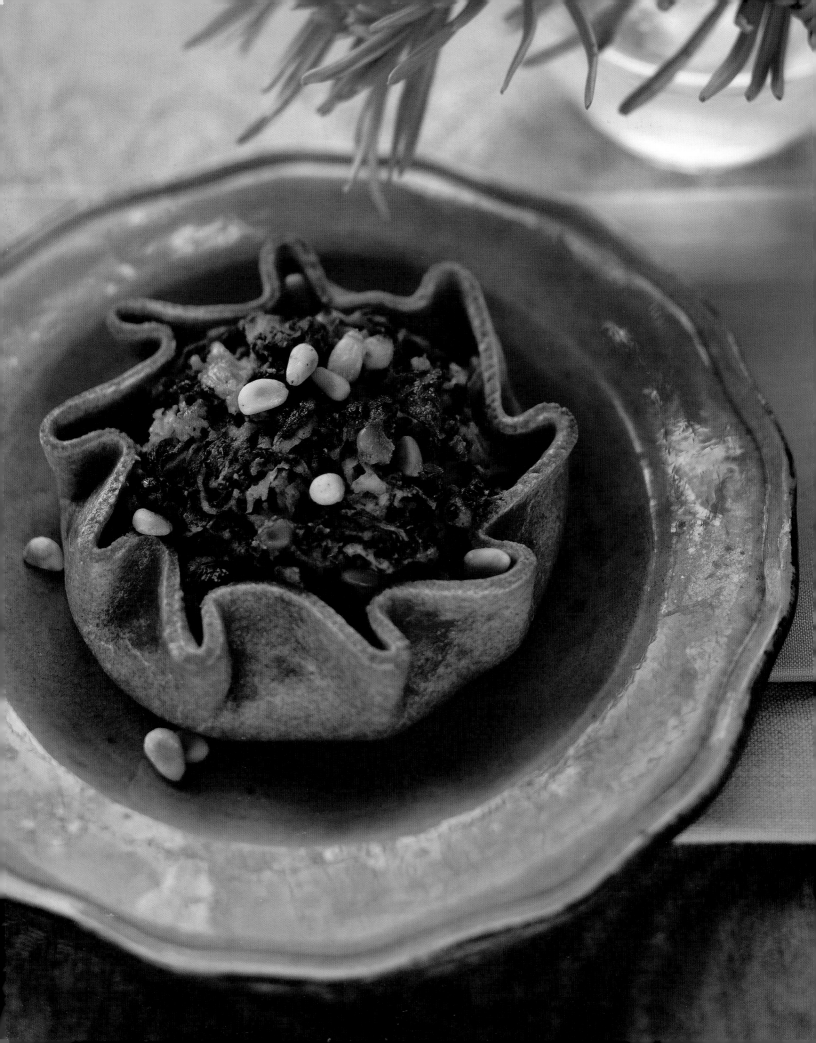

Swiss Chard "Ricotta" Galettes

This is where we go in the way-back machine to come up with another way to get tasty veggies into a meal. Spelt has been around since we were in the trees. It's the ancestor of modern wheat, and it forms the crust for this takeoff on Italian tortes. The "ricotta"—which isn't really cheese but tofu—provides extra protein. Fold in the pine nuts and raisins if you want to honor our culinary ancestors and their traditions.

FILLING

4 bunches Swiss chard (2 pounds)

2 tablespoons extra virgin olive oil

1 cup finely chopped yellow onion

Pinches of sea salt

$1/_8$ teaspoon red pepper flakes

1 tablespoon finely chopped garlic

1 recipe Herbed "Ricotta" (page 118)

1 cup dried currants

$1/_2$ cup pine nuts, lightly toasted, (see page 151) (optional)

$1/_4$ teaspoon freshly grated nutmeg

1 recipe Savory Spelt Tart Crust (page 88)

Flour, for dusting

1 organic egg, beaten in a small bowl with a fork (egg wash)

INNER COOK NOTES

Spread a layer of ricotta cheese on the bottom of the dough and top with Delicata Squash with Dino Kale and Cranberry (page 41) and assemble and bake as instructed. Or roast your favorite vegetables, add some goat cheese, and voilà! If you can't find spelt flour and want more traditional dough, try the Potpie Pastry Crust (page 70).

Clean the Swiss chard and remove the tough stems. Put the greens in a bowl of cold water for a bath, allowing the dirt and sand to fall to the bottom. Lift out and cut by roll-ing in bunches, cutting into thin ribbons, and then cutting lengthwise into small bite-size pieces. Small bites of greens are more tender and easier to digest. Return to a bowl of clean cold water until ready to use.

In a large sauté pan, heat the olive oil. Sauté the onion with a pinch of salt until golden, about 5 minutes. Add the red pepper flakes and garlic and sauté for 30 seconds, just until aromatic. Add the greens with a pinch or two of salt and cook until tender. The water that adheres to the greens will be enough to cook them. Set aside to cool. Drain and squeeze out any remaining liquid.

In a medium bowl, combine the greens with the "ricotta," currants, pine nuts, and nutmeg. Taste. Does it need a pinch of salt or a squeeze of lemon? Refrigerate until ready to use.

Preheat the oven to 375°F.

To make individual galettes, line a sheet pan with parchment paper. Cut the dough into 6 equal portions. Lightly dust your work surface with flour and roll each piece of dough into a circle about 8 inches in diameter and $1/_{16}$ inch thick or less. Spoon $1/_2$ cup of the chard mixture into the center of the crust (being careful not to overfill); leave an uncovered edge of dough at least an inch wide all the way around. Brush the edge of the circle with egg wash.

Making galettes can be a blast, especially in a group. There are so many possible fillings. One of my favorite classes involved eight women, including Andrea, a cancer survivor. The women sat in Andrea's beautiful country home. Everyone had a rolling pin. Some galettes came out fat, others were thin, and the fillings included goat cheese, leek, cherry tomatoes, onions, and more. Andrea did the Swiss chard, and she sounded pretty pleased with the results. "It was as if I left my body and mind behind and just lived inside the taste for a few precious moments."

(continued on next page)

Work your way around the galette and crimp the dough up all around the galette. Use a pastry brush or your fingers to brush the egg wash on the exposed dough. Transfer the galettes to the lined sheet pan and bake for 20 minutes, until golden brown.

To make 2 larger free-form galettes, divide the dough in half and roll each piece to approximately 12 inches in diameter and $1/16$ inch thick. Follow the instructions above and bake for 25 to 30 minutes.

Makes 6 individual galettes or 2 large galettes (Serves 6)

PER SERVING Calories: 486; Total Fat: 23 g (3 g saturated, 13 g monounsaturated); Carbohydrates: 60 g; Protein: 14 g; Fiber: 10 g; Sodium: 777 mg

Savory Spelt Tart Crust

$1^1/4$ cups whole wheat pastry flour

1 cup organic spelt flour

2 teaspoons baking powder

$1/2$ teaspoon sea salt

$1/4$ cup extra virgin olive oil

$1/2$ cup water

1 teaspoon maple syrup

In a food processor fitted with the metal blade, process both flours, baking powder, and salt for about 10 seconds to mix. Whisk together the olive oil, water, and maple syrup and pour over the flour mixture. Pulse until just blended. Gather together the dough and divide it into six parts if making individual galettes or two if making a large pie. Form the dough into round, flat disks. Wrap in plastic wrap and refrigerate for at least 30 minutes.

Makes 6 individual galettes, or two 12-inch rounds (Serves 6)

PER SERVING Calories: 240; Total Fat: 10 g (1 g saturated, 6 g monounsaturated); Carbohydrates: 32 g; Protein: 5 g; Fiber: 5 g; Sodium: 429 mg

INNER COOK NOTES

Spelt is the grandmother of wheat. It contains less gluten, and therefore is easier to digest. You can use all spelt flour in this recipe, but the texture will be a bit denser. If you really want to be adventurous, try using sprouted flours. The sprouting of the grains makes them even easier to digest and more flavorful. Look in the Resource Guide in the back for tips on where to find these special ingredients.

Ginger Brown Basmati Rice

This rice has a nutty, aromatic taste, but it's the ginger that carries the day. Ginger fires up your stomach's digestive enzymes. This makes the dish light on the constitution and ensures maximum absorption of nutrients. The Culinary Terms of Endearment chapter explains the benefits of soaking rice. Soaked brown rice usually cooks in half the time of rice that hasn't been soaked.

$^1/_2$ teaspoon sea salt

1 (2 by 1-inch) piece of kombu

1 (1-inch slice) unpeeled fresh ginger

1 cup brown basmati rice, soaked overnight with 2 cups water and the juice and rind of $^1/_2$ lemon

In a 2-quart pot, bring $2^1/_2$ cups of water to a boil over high heat. Add the salt, kombu, ginger, and rice (remember to rinse it well after its overnight spa). Return to a boil. Decrease the heat, cover, and simmer for 20 to 25 minutes. Check the rice at 20 minutes; if there are steam holes on the top, it's ready. Fluff with a fork and serve.

Serves 6

PER SERVING Calories: 107; Total Fat: 1 g (0 g saturated, 0 g monounsaturated); Carbohydrates: 23 g; Protein: 2 g; Fiber: 2 g; Sodium: 208 mg

INNER COOK NOTES
Some people think of sea vegetables as slimy. Slimy is most people's least favorite texture. Serving something slimy is worse than telling your children they have to eat their spinach. However, kombu is a magical sea vegetable. It can be hidden in soups, a pot of beans, or rice. During the cooking process, it releases all of its powerful, healing mineral content into the liquid. When the cooking is done, you can discard the kombu—without having to deal with its slimy texture. Now you see it—now you don't.

Garlicky Brown Basmati Rice

$^1/_2$ teaspoon sea salt

1 (2 by 1-inch) piece of kombu

1 clove garlic, smashed

1 cup brown basmati rice, soaked overnight with 2 cups water and the juice and rind of $^1/_2$ lemon

In a 2-quart pot, bring $2^1/_2$ cups of water to a boil over high heat. Add the salt, kombu, garlic, and rice (remember to rinse it well after its overnight spa). Return to a boil. Decrease the heat, cover, and simmer for 20 to 25 minutes. Check the rice at 20 minutes; if there are steam holes on the top, it's ready. Fluff with a fork and serve.

Serves 6

PER SERVING Calories: 107; Total Fat: 1 g (0 g saturated, 0 g monounsaturated); Carbohydrates: 23 g; Protein: 2 g; Fiber: 2 g; Sodium: 208 mg

Asian Japonica Rice Salad with Edamame

For ages, buying rice in America was like walking into an ice cream store and finding they had only two flavors. The vanilla of the rice world is bleached white rice, which has had its nutrients strip-mined away. Its chocolate counterpart is tasteless short-grain brown rice, which gave rise to the phrase "hippie gruel." Fortunately, many different types of rice are now available—basmati, jasmine, sushi rice. . . . Japonica is a terrific choice for rice salads because of its nutty taste and firm texture.

2 teaspoons sea salt

2 cups black Japonica rice, rinsed and drained

1 cup shelled edamame beans

1 cup peeled and thinly sliced diagonally celery

1 cup peeled and shredded carrot

$^1/_2$ red bell pepper, diced

$^1/_2$ cup thinly sliced diagonally scallions, green and white parts

DRESSING

2 tablespoons brown rice vinegar

3 tablespoons tamari

1 tablespoon minced fresh ginger

2 cloves garlic, minced

$^1/_8$ teaspoon cayenne

$^1/_4$ cup sesame oil

1 teaspoon toasted sesame oil

3 tablespoons fresh lime juice

$^1/_8$ teaspoon sea salt

$^1/_2$ teaspoon maple syrup

1 cup toasted cashews (see page 151)

1 tablespoon chopped fresh cilantro

$^1/_2$ cup chopped fresh basil

1 tablespoon lightly toasted sesame seeds (see page 151)

2 teaspoons fresh lime juice

In a medium pot, bring 4 cups of water and 1 teaspoon salt to a boil over high heat. Add the rice and return to a boil. Cover, decrease the heat, and simmer until tender, 40 to 45 minutes. Pour the rice onto a sheet pan and fluff with a fork to separate the grains and cool.

In another medium pot, bring 4 cups of water to a boil over high heat. Add 1 teaspoon salt and blanch the edamame until just tender, about 1 minute. Transfer to a colander, rinse with cold water, and set aside.

In a bowl combine the rice, celery, carrot, red pepper, and scallions. Prepare the dressing by whisking the vinegar, tamari, ginger, garlic, cayenne, sesame oil, toasted sesame oil, lime juice, salt, and maple syrup together. Toss the rice mixture with the dressing. Stir in the beans, cashews (reserve a few for garnish), cilantro, and basil. Top with the sesame seeds and a squeeze of lime juice. Serve in a salad bowl, garnished with cashews.

Serves 8

PER SERVING Calories: 393; Total Fat: 18 g (3 g saturated, 8 g monounsaturated); Carbohydrates: 50 g; Protein: 11 g; Fiber: 6 g; Sodium: 811 mg

The Big O: It seems strange that an unassuming food like celery would have such a celebrated history: Celery tonics were once touted as cure-alls for ailments ranging from gout to hangovers. As with most folk remedies, there's a touch of truth behind the myths, and several good reasons to seek out organic sources. Celery's high water content and ability to relax arterial walls suggests it interacts with the body extensively, which means you might want to avoid conventionally grown celery as it tends to be heavily treated with pesticides.

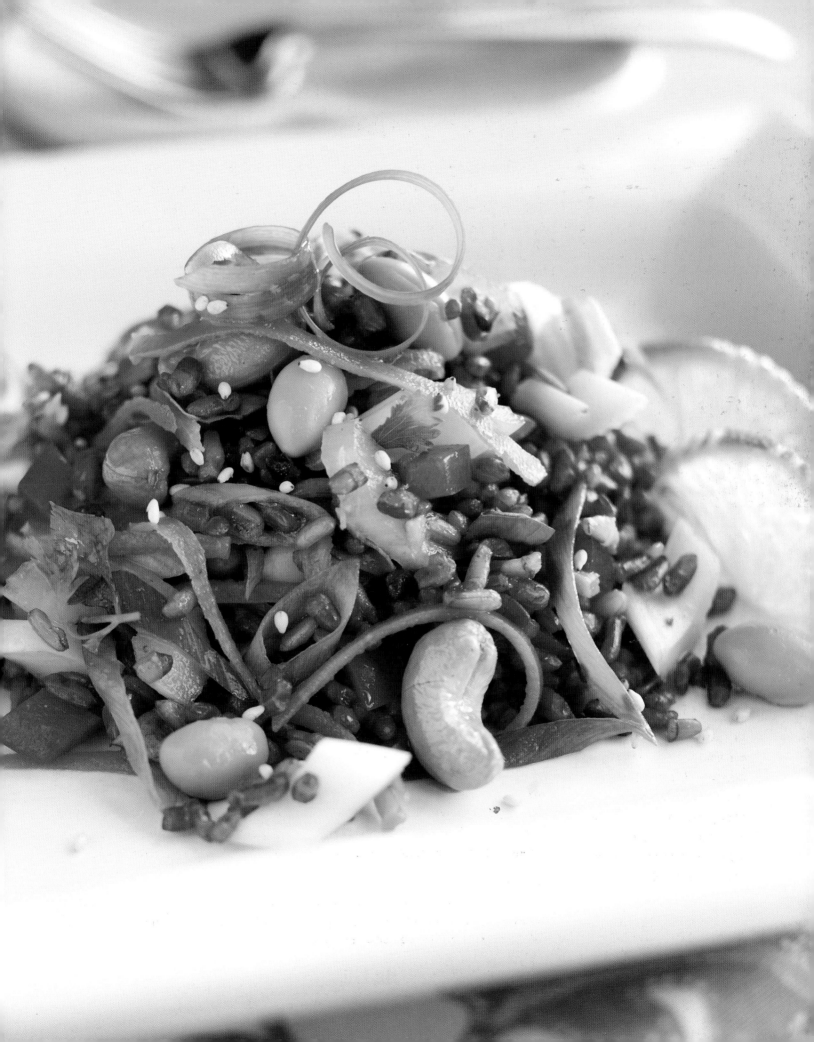

Cornmeal Pizza

This is a great example of a creative way to hide greens. One of my clients knew she needed to eat greens, but she really couldn't face them head-on. The answer? Put them on a pizza. No one I know is immune to pizza's siren call, probably because it's so easy to customize to taste. Pesto, tomato sauce, dark greens, olives, feta, goat cheese . . . the variations are endless. The cornmeal crust pulls everything together: it won't get soggy even if the pizza is stored in the fridge or freezer. As a pie, it makes a meal for family and friends. By the slice, it's a perfect companion for salads or soups.

1 package of 2 Vicolo cornmeal crusts

$^{1}/_{2}$ cup prepared chunky tomato sauce or pesto

Topping options (see note)

$^{1}/_{4}$ cup grated organic Parmesan or crumbled organic goat cheese (optional)

Kalamata olives or your favorite olives

Preheat the oven to 425°F.

Bake the pizza crusts for about 5 minutes, or until golden brown. Remove from the oven and build your pizzas. Start with tomato sauce or pesto, add vegetables, and top with cheese and olives. Bake for 15 minutes, or until the toppings are bubbly and the cheese is melted. Serve hot with a mixed green salad.

Serves 6

PER SERVING Calories: 351; Total Fat: 15 g (0 g saturated, 0 g monounsaturated); Carbohydrates: 43 g; Protein: 7 g; Fiber: 1 g; Sodium: 476 mg

Frittata with Herby Potatoes

Frittatas are like a quiche without a crust. They're a classic Italian egg combination, amenable to just about any vegetable you can conjure up. People sensitive to temperature like frittatas because they can be served lukewarm or at room temperature. Eggs are also a great source of protein. Mix in a little Simon and Garfunkel—parsley, sage, rosemary, and thyme—and a filling frittata becomes an anytime classic.

INNER COOK NOTES
Be creative; most vegetables will taste great in this frittata. Try the following combinations: cherry tomatoes, spinach, and feta; zucchini, yellow crook-neck squash, and basil; and caramelized onions. Create away!

FILLING

1 tablespoon extra virgin olive oil

2 tablespoons finely chopped shallot, onion, or fennel

$^1/_2$ cup diced small red potatoes

Pinches of sea salt

$1^1/_4$ teaspoons dried thyme

$^1/_8$ teaspoon freshly ground pepper

Pinch of cayenne

EGGS

8 large organic eggs

$^1/_4$ cup low-fat organic milk or soy milk

Pinch of sea salt

$1^1/_2$ teaspoons dried herbs (a combination of thyme, marjoram, and basil)

$^1/_8$ teaspoon freshly grated nutmeg

Pinch of freshly ground pepper

Pinch of cayenne

$^1/_4$ cup asparagus, tough stems removed, peeled, and cut into bite-size pieces

$^1/_4$ cup freshly grated organic Parmesan or Monterey Jack cheese, or 2 ounces organic goat cheese, crumbled (optional)

Preheat the oven to 325°F. Lightly oil an 8-inch glass pie pan or 8-inch square glass baking dish.

In a large sauté pan, heat the olive oil over medium heat. Add the shallot and cook until just soft. Add the potatoes and a pinch of salt and sauté until brown and crispy. Add the thyme, another pinch of salt, the pepper, and cayenne. Stir to thoroughly coat.

Whisk the eggs, milk, a pinch of salt, herb mixture, nutmeg, pepper, and cayenne in a medium bowl with a balloon whisk. You are really whisking now, not just breaking up the eggs, but whisking them well until foamy. No cheating; whisk at least 30 times.

Add the potato mixture, asparagus, and cheese to the eggs and stir to combine. Pour into the prepared pan. Bake for 20 to 25 minutes, or until the edges are pulling away from the side and the center is firm to the touch or "jiggle free". Let cool for about 5 minutes. Run a knife around the edge to loosen and cut into wedges. Serve warm or at room temperature.

Serves 6

PER SERVING Calories: 137; Total Fat: 9 g (2 g saturated, 4 g monounsaturated); Carbohydrates: 5 g; Protein: 9 g; Fiber: 1 g; Sodium: 173 mg

The key to making a frittata is whipping the eggs into a froth. In Italy the *signoras* know if you're capable of this by looking at your whisking forearm. They frown if it isn't twice the size of your other forearm. My trick is to count to thirty.

The Big O: Why should you go organic with eggs? Oh, let me count the ways. The organic feed that organic layers consume produces eggs rich in minerals and taste. The yolks are a plump deep orange-yellow, the whites clearer and less runny . . . in all, organic eggs blow everything else off the shelf. When shopping for them, look for brands labeled "Omega-3." This means they've come from chickens fed flaxseed, which further enriches the nutritional value of their eggs.

Ginger Ale with Grape Cubes

INNER COOK NOTES
Ginger root's healing properties are well-documented in the scientific literature: motion sickness, morning sickness, and nausea associated with chemotherapy and surgery all appear to be lessened by consumption of a little ginger.

The frozen grapes will keep for up to 3 months in an airtight container.

The Big O: For kids, consuming organic grapes are especially important. An EPA report noted that, of all fruits, conventionally grown grapes "emerged as a major risk-driver" of childhood health problems because those grapes are grown with an insecticide that blocks a body enzyme, cholinesterase, vital for proper nervous system function.

INNER COOK NOTES
For a change, try making this recipe with chamomile and ginger blend organic tea bags.

Why would you make your own ginger ale when there are twenty-four varieties in the supermarket? For the same reason people make their own iced tea. Canned and bottled ginger ales generally have a ton of refined sugar. Also, the ginger they contain is so diluted that its taste is barely discernible. That's not the case when you make it yourself, which is surprisingly easy to do. You can vary the strength of the ginger syrup, all the while knowing that in this form ginger can soothe and aid digestion.

2 cups sliced, unpeeled fresh ginger	Organic seedless grapes, frozen in a sealed plastic bag
2 tablespoons fresh lemon juice	Sparkling water
2 tablespoons organic honey	Fresh mint sprigs, for garnish

Place 4 cups of water and the ginger in a saucepan and bring to a boil over high heat. Reduce the heat and simmer, covered, for 1 hour. Uncover and continue to simmer for 30 minutes. Strain through cheesecloth. Stir in the lemon juice and honey, cool to room temperature and store in the refrigerator for up to 1 week.

For a cold drink, add $1/4$ cup of syrup to a glass of grape cubes and fill the glass with sparkling water. Garnish with a sprig of mint. For a hot drink, add 3 tablespoons of the syrup to a cup of hot water. Adjust with additional honey or lemon, if needed.

Makes about 2 cups syrup

PER SERVING Calories: 36; Total Fat: 0 g (0 g saturated, 0 g monounsaturated); Carbohydrates: 9 g; Protein: 0 g; Fiber: 1 g; Sodium: 3 mg

Ginger Tea

3 organic ginger tea bags	$1/4$ teaspoon fresh lemon juice
$1/4$ teaspoon honey	Sparkling water

Pour 2 cups boiling water over the tea bags and steep for 15 minutes. Pour into a small saucepan and reduce by half over medium heat. Stir in the honey and lemon juice. Cool to room temperature and store in the refrigerator for up to 1 week. To serve, add 2 tablespoons of the ginger syrup to your favorite glass and add sparkling water.

Makes 1 cup

PER SERVING Calories: 1; Total Fat: 0 g (0 g saturated, 0 g monounsaturated); Carbohydrates: 0 g; Protein: 0 g; Fiber: 0 g; Sodium: 2 mg

Pecans Spiced with Orange Zest and Ginger

Sometimes you feel like a nut. Sometimes you feel like a really tasty *nut. That's when you reach for these bad boys. Actually they're not bad at all. Just addictive. Precisely the right amount of sweet, spice (that's the ginger), and yum. They smell good, too. Eat them alone or crumbled over salads or greens. Go nuts!*

2 tablespoons orange zest (zest of 1 large orange)

1/4 teaspoon sea salt

1 tablespoon maple syrup

2 teaspoons extra virgin olive oil

Pinch of red pepper flakes

1/4 teaspoon grated fresh ginger

2 cups pecan halves

Preheat the oven to 350°F.

Combine the zest, salt, maple syrup, olive oil, red pepper flakes, and ginger in a small bowl and whisk until well blended.

Put the pecans in a resealable plastic bag and pour in the coating mixture. Push all the air out of the bag, seal it, and squeeze the pecans around inside the bag until they are well coated. Pour in a single layer on a sheet pan and bake for about 12 minutes, until you can smell them!

Remove from the oven and cool to room temperature. The nuts will become crispy as they cool. Loosen from the sheet pan with a metal spatula and take a bite!

Makes 2 cups (Serves 6)

PER SERVING Calories: 50; Total Fat: 10 g; (0 g saturated, 6 g monounsaturated); Carbohydrates: 12 g; Protein: 0 g; Fiber: 1 g; Sodium: 6 mg

INNER COOK NOTES
Pecans don't float your boat? Try almonds or walnuts instead.

Anytime you zest a fruit—which means removing the colorful rind of the fruit with a fine grater—wash it thoroughly first. After all, you never know who's been fondling your fruit.

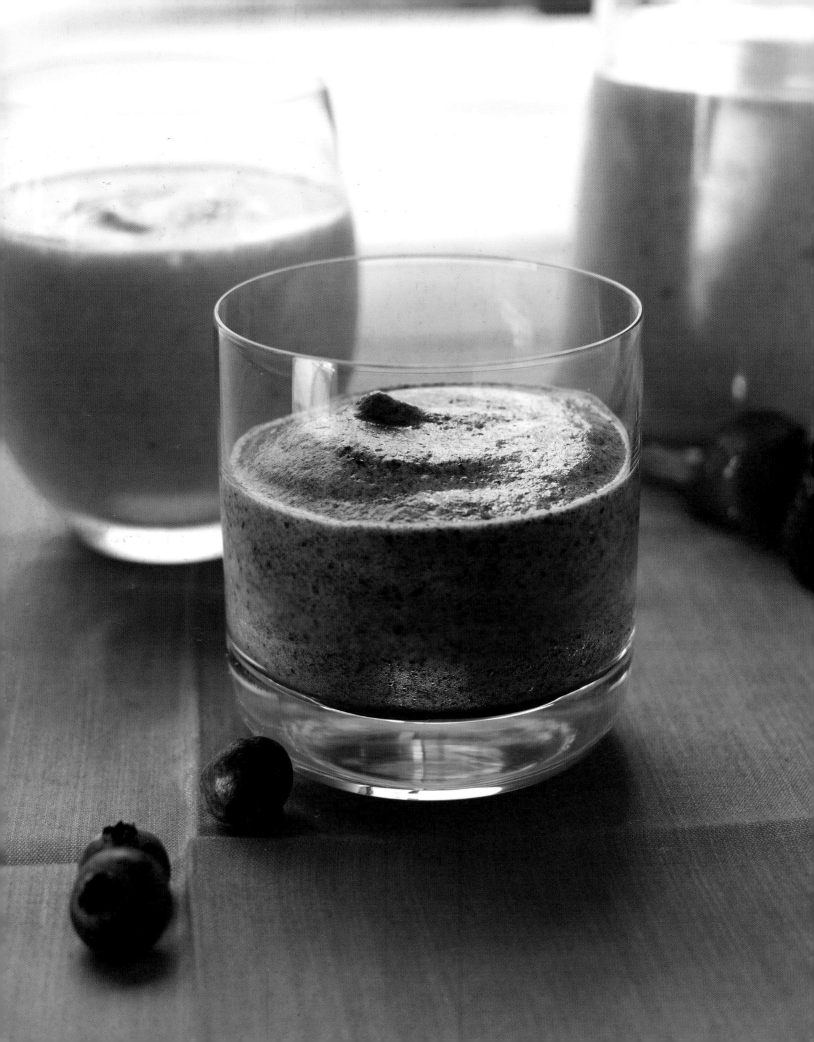

Blueberry Slush Smoothie

Smoothies can be a best friend to someone in the middle of cancer treatments. They're a cool, creamy, sweet meal in a glass. I like that smoothies can be kept in the refrigerator and sipped over the course of a day. I often dole smoothies out in shot glasses, as some of my clients don't want more than 2 ounces at a time. That's still enough liquid to contain a nutritional punch, thanks to a dash of whey protein powder and ground flax seed. The blueberry slush is the lighter of the two smoothies. It can be easily sipped through a straw.

1 cup frozen blueberries

$^1/_2$ cup lemon Recharge or fruit juice

1 "whey scoop" of whey protein powder

1 tablespoon ground flax seed

6 ice cubes

Combine the blueberries, Recharge, protein powder, flax seed, and ice cubes with $^1/_2$ cup water in a blender and purée. You have a light, frothy drink packed with protein! Pour into a beautiful glass.

Makes about 20 ounces (Serves 5)

PER SERVING Calories: 51; Total Fat: 1 g (0 g saturated, 0 g monounsaturated); Carbohydrates: 6 g; Protein: 5 g; Fiber: 1 g; Sodium: 9 mg

Flax seed should be handled with kid gloves. The oils they contain are very sensitive to heat and can quickly turn rancid. I suggest buying small quantities of the seed instead of flax seed oil. Store it whole in the freezer and pulverize it in a grinder when ready for use. The seed provides essential fatty acids that reduce inflammation that may be associated with certain cancers and heart disease. If you're not putting flax in a smoothie, sprinkle some over oatmeal or a salad.

Creamy Banana-Coconut Shake

This thick and creamy smoothie has the texture of a milkshake.

1 (5.5-ounce) can coconut milk	1 tablespoon ground flax seed
1 medium-size ripe banana	Pinch of sea salt
$1/_2$ cup frozen strawberries	Spritz of fresh lemon juice
1 "whey scoop" of whey protein powder	6 ice cubes

Combine the coconut milk, banana, strawberries, protein powder, flax seed, salt, lemon juice, and ice cubes with 5 tablespoons water in a blender and purée. Not only do you have velvet covering your taste buds, but put it in the freezer for an hour and voilà! Frozen yogurt.

Makes about 20 ounces (Serves 5)

PER SERVING Calories: 148; Total Fat: 9 g (7 g saturated, 0 g monounsaturated); Carbohydrates: 10 g; Protein: 8 g; Fiber: 2 g; Sodium: 54 mg

The Big O: Strawberries always seem to be such fragile little fruits, and now I know why. According to the Environmental Working Group, a science-based non-profit, the commercially grown strawberry has one of the highest concentrations of chemical compounds. That's too many devils dancing on the head of a pin! Organically grown or unsprayed berries are smaller and have more intense color, which means more antioxidants. Bite for bite, they are sweeter and more nutrient dense than their conventional counterparts. Keep in mind that you can buy organic strawberries in season and freeze them to use in smoothies.

Pita Crisps with Parmesan and Variations on the Theme

See ya', Doritos. Here's a simple, healthy munchie that's easy to make. All it takes is a few pitas cut into triangles. Using olive oil or a little Parmesan, these basic bites can be jazzed up with cumin, cayenne, or oregano. Alone, with dip, or as an accompaniment to a meal, these crisps are a fantastic all-purpose snack.

1 package small pita breads (8 to 10 pieces)

Freshly grated organic Parmesan cheese, for sprinkling

Preheat the oven to 350°F. Cut the pita breads into quarters and split the layers. Arrange the quarters in a single layer on sheet pans. Sprinkle with the Parmesan and bake until crisp and the cheese melts, 8 to 10 minutes. Serve in a bowl with some of your favorite dollops!

Makes 30 to 40 (Serves 6)

PER SERVING Calories: 210; Total Fat: 3 g (1 g saturated, 0 g monounsaturated); Carbohydrates: 36 g; Protein: 9 g; Fiber: 5 g; Sodium: 483 mg

> **INNER COOK NOTES**
> Use a pastry brush to lightly brush the pita with olive oil and sprinkle with oregano. Bake for 8 to 10 minutes, until golden. Remove from the oven and cool. Stores well in an airtight container for up to 1 week.
>
> Use the same process for flour tortillas, brushing them with oil and sprinkling with crushed cumin seeds to serve with the Tortilla Stack with Salsa Cruda (page 62), Avocado Cream (page 115), or Black Bean Medley (page 85).

Spiced Roasted Almonds

People always ask me what's the best snack to have when they're at work, stuck in traffic, or just in that never-never land between lunch and dinner. My answer often surprises them: roasted almonds. Almonds, though tiny, are a superfood, full of nutrients and proteins, and—for those hypoglycemic moments—able to balance your blood sugar. They also help reduce sugar and salt cravings.

2 cups organic raw almonds

1 teaspoon extra virgin olive oil

$1/2$ teaspoon sea salt

Pinch of cayenne

Preheat the oven to 350°F. Toss the almonds, olive oil, salt, and cayenne in a large mixing bowl until the almonds are coated. Spread in a single layer on a sheet pan. Bake for 10 to 15 minutes, or until the almonds turn golden brown. You know they're done when you can smell them.

Remove from the oven and cool. The nuts will become crispy as they cool.

Makes 2 cups (Serves 16)

PER SERVING Calories: 108; Total Fat: 10 g (0 g saturated, 6 g monounsaturated); Carbohydrates: 3 g; Protein: 4 g; Fiber: 2 g; Sodium: 74 mg

> **INNER COOK NOTES**
> Nuts can be stored in an airtight container in your freezer for 6 months. When you're ready to eat them, put them in a bowl and allow them to come to room temperature.
>
> Toast a sheet of nori by waving it over a flame two or three times and cut it into small bite-size pieces. Mix in with the almonds when cooled. Or, for a sweeter treat, toss in $1/4$ cup dried cranberries while the nuts are still warm.

Coconut-Ginger Rice with Cilantro

INNER COOK NOTES
This is a great recipe to double so you have leftovers. Use a large can of coconut milk (sizes vary from 12 to 15 ounces) and adjust the quantity of water and the remaining ingredients.

Not everyone likes cilantro. If that includes you, substitute a little chopped fresh flat-leaf parsley or chopped fresh mint, or just skip the herbs entirely. The dish will still be delicious.

Jen took a batch of this rice to her support group and they went bananas. Jen's friend told her that her kids didn't even realize they were eating brown rice. One small step for Mom . . .

I wish I had a nice, shiny nickel for every client who has said to me, "Rebecca, I'm trying to eat well, but I am soooooo sick of boring brown rice." My friend Jen went through this as she was recovering from breast cancer; her family threatened mutiny if they saw plain brown rice one more time. I told her, "Honey, do I have a recipe for you!" Coconut milk softens and sweetens the generally grainy, tasteless brown rice. The cilantro, so familiar to fans of Thai food, provides a fresh high note.

1 (5.5-ounce) can coconut milk

1 teaspoon sea salt

1 inch unpeeled fresh ginger, thinly sliced into rounds

1 cup brown jasmine or basmati rice, rinsed until the water runs clear

$1/4$ cup coarsely chopped fresh cilantro

In a pot with a tight-fitting lid, combine the coconut milk, $1^1/4$ cups water, and the salt. Smash the ginger pieces with the flat side of your knife to release their flavor and add them to the pot. Bring to a rolling boil over medium heat. Add the rice and stir well. Return the water to a boil, cover, and decrease the heat to low. Simmer for 20 minutes, until the water is fully absorbed.

Remove the pot from the heat and let stand, covered, for about 10 minutes. Uncover and remove and discard the ginger. Add the cilantro and gently toss with a fork. Serve in individual bowls or in a colorful serving bowl.

Serves 6

PER SERVING Calories: 165; Total Fat: 6 g (5 g saturated, 0 g monounsaturated); Carbohydrates: 24 g; Protein: 3 g; Fiber: 1 g; Sodium: 396 mg

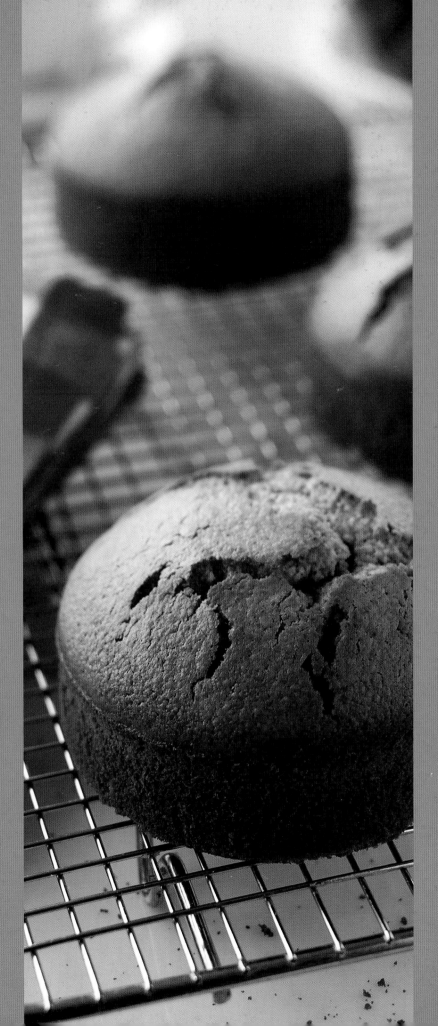

I'm a pragmatist at heart. A lot of people with cancer have heard that they should forgo sweets because refined sugar is bad, bad, bad for them. Yet cancer treatments can often increase the craving for sweets, especially for people who find they have a bitter or metallic taste in their mouth. I've seen some of these folks swear off sugar as long as they can, then go off on a Ding Dong binge.

NOT A GOOD THING. I've tried to come up with a better approach. The sweet bites you'll find in this chapter all have one thing in common: they contain no refined sugar. There are so many better, healthier ways to get a sweet taste. A small amount of organic Grade B maple syrup is enough to sweeten these bites, which also use fruits, nuts, oats, and some surprise ingredients (coconut oil!) to pump up the yum.

As my grandmother would say, everything in moderation, including moderation. Whether it's the Gingerbread (page 111), the Almond Chocolate Chip Cookies (opposite), the Fruit Parfait (page 112), or any of these recipes, you'll find they're so rich that just a morsel will indulge and quell those sweet cravings. And we've even filled those normally empty calories with lots of nutrition. Bet you didn't think you could find a sweet treat that was so good for you to eat!

Almond Chocolate Chip Cookies

This recipe was born of desperation. I had a client struggling with his appetite. He was losing weight and had completely lost his connection with food, with one exception: he loved chocolate chip cookies. Of course, the cookies he ate were full of refined sugar and empty calories. Instead of fruitlessly arguing with him or nagging him to eat "better" foods, I figured it made more sense to meet him where he was most comfortable. I came up with these cookies, which contain no dairy or refined sugar. The only question was whether my client would like the taste. He took one bite and a huge smile spread across his face.

$1/2$ cup finely chopped blanched or raw almonds, pulsed in a food processor to form small granules

2 cups organic all-purpose unbleached flour or organic spelt flour

1 teaspoon aluminum-free baking powder

$1/2$ teaspoon baking soda

$1/4$ teaspoon sea salt

1 cup dark chocolate chips

$1/2$ cup melted coconut oil

$1/2$ cup maple syrup

1 teaspoon vanilla extract

INNER COOK NOTES
Once cooled, these cookies can be frozen in airtight containers for 2 months. Take out a few and warm in a toaster oven for 5 minutes at 350°F for that fresh-baked bite.

If you prefer, try walnuts or, if you're feeling decadent, macadamia nuts. Don't worry if your doctor has said to pass on nuts. This recipe also works without them.

Preheat the oven to 350°F. Line a baking sheet with parchment paper.

In a large bowl, combine the pulsed almonds, flour, baking powder, baking soda, salt, and chocolate chips.

In a small bowl, whisk together the coconut oil, maple syrup, vanilla extract, and $1/2$ cup water. Pour into the dry ingredients. With a spatula, mix the dough until very well combined.

Form cookies by placing 1 tablespoon of dough at a time on the prepared baking sheet. Use a spoon to flatten the tops. Bake for 8 to 10 minutes. The cookies are done when the bottoms are deep golden brown and the tops are lightly brown. Transfer to a rack and cool.

Makes 30 cookies

PER SERVING Calories: 119; Total Fat: 7 g (4 g saturated, 0 g monounsaturated); Carbohydrates: 15 g; Protein: 2 g; Fiber: 1 g; Sodium: 56 mg

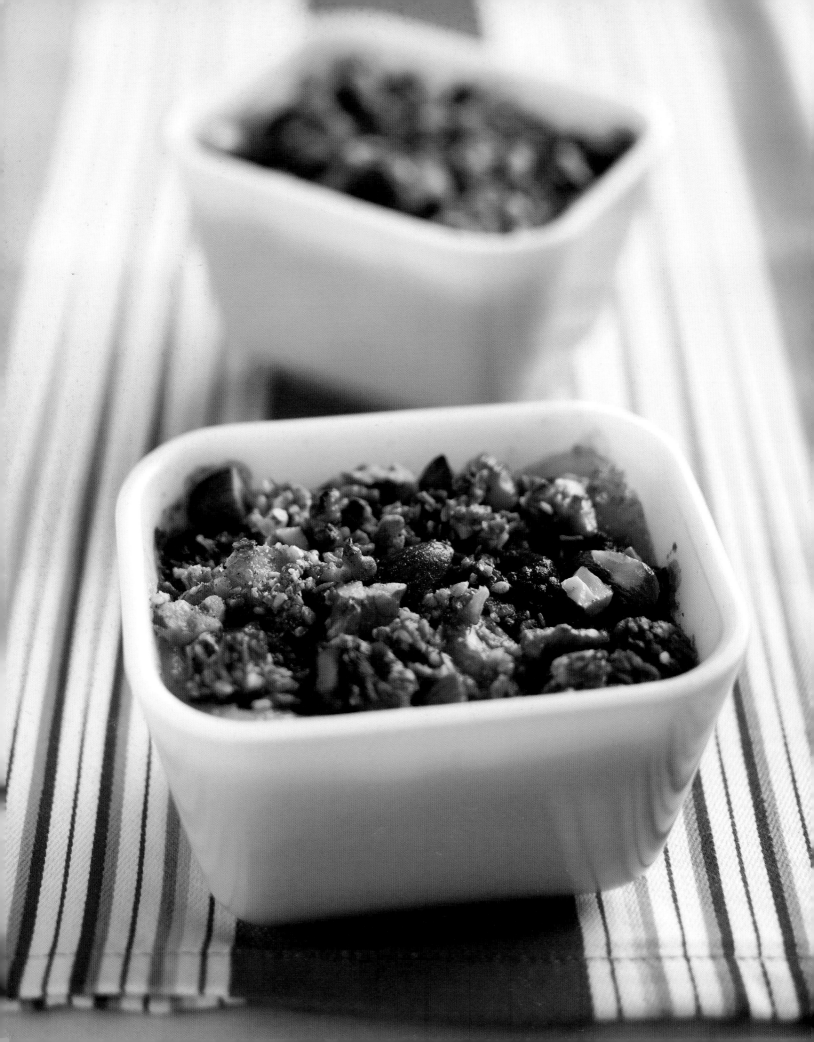

Fruit Crisp

I chanced into this recipe while cooking at Commonweal. For some reason, we had an abundance of berries in the kitchen. I took one look at the weather—it was a cold, damp morning—and decided it was time to have some fun with breakfast. I looked back at the berries, glanced over at a bowl of mixed nuts on a countertop, and saw a possibility. The berries got tossed with some spices, the mixed nuts got pulsed in the food processor, and the makeshift crisp went into the oven. Within minutes the kitchen smelled like a bubbling berry bonanza. Did it work? Put it this way: An hour later, the pie plate came back to the kitchen clean as a whistle.

INNER COOK NOTES
Any fruit—raspberries, peaches, apples, or a combination—can be used. And if you don't have time to make the Anytime Crunch, use granola or a hearty healthy cereal.

1 teaspoon kudzu root powder

$2^2/_3$ cups organic fresh or frozen blueberries (2 10-ounce bags)

$1/_2$ teaspoon powdered ginger

$1/_2$ teaspoon ground cinnamon

$1/_4$ teaspoon ground cardamom

1 tablespoon fresh lemon juice

2 tablespoons maple syrup or other organic sweetener

$1/_8$ teaspoon sea salt

3 cups Anytime Crunch (page 83), pulsed briefly in the food processor

Preheat the oven to 350°F. Lightly oil or butter a 9-inch glass pie plate or 9-inch square baking dish.

In a small bowl, dissolve the kudzu in 2 tablespoons of cold water. In a large bowl, combine the blueberries, ginger, cinnamon, cardamom, lemon juice, maple syrup, salt, and kudzu slurry. Let the fruit sit for about 15 minutes so the spices are absorbed. Pour into the prepared baking dish, top with the Anytime Crunch, and use a large spoon to pat the topping down into the fruit. Bake for 25 minutes, or until bubbly. Cool for about 15 minutes. Serve in small bowls warm or at room temperature.

Serves 8

PER SERVING Calories: 500; Total Fat: 34 g (3 g saturated, 6 g monounsaturated); Carbohydrates: 43 g; Protein: 12 g; Fiber: 9 g; Sodium: 85 mg

Cashew Tart Crusts with Fresh Berries

I love using cashews in this dessert because it results in a buttery crust without even a smidge of butter. These crusts are also much healthier than the tart crusts that populate most supermarket shelves, which are high in trans fats. The dough doesn't need to be beaten into submission with a rolling pin; simply press it into a tart pan with your fingers. This crust's uses are limited only by your imagination. This version has a small amount of goat cheese as a base for fresh strawberries and blueberries. The crust is also so rich that a little slice of whatever you decide to put in will be very satiating.

1 cup raw cashews

$1/2$ cup Spectrum unrefined expeller-pressed safflower oil

$1/4$ cup maple syrup

$1/2$ teaspoon sea salt

$1/2$ teaspoon aluminum-free baking powder

$1^3/4$ cups organic unbleached all-purpose flour

$1/4$ cup organic goat cheese, mascarpone, or farmer's cheese, at room temperature

1 teaspoon fresh lemon juice

$1/4$ teaspoon grated lemon zest

$1/4$ teaspoon maple syrup

2 cups stemmed and sliced fresh strawberries

$1/4$ cup fresh blueberries

Preheat the oven to 350°F. Line the bottom of a tart pan with parchment paper.

In a food processor fitted with a metal blade, process the cashews to a fine texture, about 1 minute. Scrape down the sides of the bowl with a spatula as necessary. With the food processor running, add the oil, maple syrup, salt, and baking powder. Process for about 1 minute. Scrape down the sides, add the flour, and process until a ball starts to form.

Transfer the dough to a large bowl. Knead the mixture with your hands until the flour is fully incorporated. If the mixture is too dry, add a few drops of water.

Press the dough in one 12-inch, two 8-inch, or six 4-inch tart pans. Fill the shells with pie weights and bake for 10 minutes. Remove the weights and continue to bake for another 5 to 10 minutes, or until golden.

In a small bowl, combine the cheese, lemon juice and zest, and maple syrup. Combine well and set aside. When the tart crust has cooled, spread a thin layer of the cheese mixture on the bottom of the tart crust. Be careful not to get too close to the edge; it may crumble. Top the cheese layer with overlapping concentric circles of strawberries and sprinkle the blueberries on top. Chill for several hours before serving. Serve in small wedges.

Makes one 12-inch, two 8-inch, or six 4-inch tart crusts (Serves 8)

PER SERVING Calories: 408; Total Fat: 29 g; (6 g saturated, 15 g monounsaturated); Carbohydrates: 35 g; Protein: 7 g; Fiber: 2 g; Sodium: 186 mg

---

INNER COOK NOTES

Pie weights can be anything from half a bag of rice or dried beans to metal weights purchased at a cookware store. Cut an oversized piece of parchment paper, lay it over the tart dough, and add your weights. Leave enough overhang of paper so you can easily lift the weights out halfway through the baking process. Pie weights prevent the tart from shrinking and puffing up on the bottom. Speaking from experience, don't skip this step.

Almonds can be substituted for the cashews. When using almonds, decrease the flour to $1^1/2$ cups. You can also substitute hazelnuts, pecans, walnuts, and pine nuts for the cashews.

For a nondairy treat try Fruit Parfait (page 112) or Sweet "Ricotta" (page 123), also topped with berries. Or sauté some currants, diced apple, and diced pear until tender and add them to the crust. Chill for several hours and serve.

Legal Cookies

I hate when the sugar police come knocking at my door. I came up with these cookies to keep them away. They're a variation on the thumbprint cookies many of us made with Mom as kids. They're legal because we've replaced the sugar with Grade B organic maple syrup and spices. These cookies provide just enough sweet to satisfy.

1 cup organic raw almonds (whole or slivered)

1 cup rolled oats

1 cup organic, unbleached all-purpose or spelt flour

$1/4$ teaspoon ground cinnamon

$1/4$ teaspoon grated fresh ginger, or $1/8$ teaspoon powdered ginger

$1/8$ teaspoon ground cardamom

$1/8$ teaspoon freshly grated nutmeg

$1/4$ teaspoon sea salt

$1/2$ cup safflower oil

$1/2$ cup maple syrup

$1/4$ teaspoon vanilla extract

Jam, for filling

Preheat the oven to 350°F. Line a baking sheet with parchment paper.

In a food processor fitted with a metal blade, grind the almonds into coarse flour, about 2 minutes. Add the oats, flour, cinnamon, ginger, cardamom, nutmeg, and salt and process for another minute.

Add the oil, maple syrup, and vanilla extract. Continue to process until well combined. The dough will quickly form into a ball. Wrap the dough in plastic wrap and let rest at room temperature for 15 minutes.

Form 1 tablespoon of dough into a ball, place on the prepared baking sheet, and make a thumb imprint in the center of each cookie. Fill with your favorite organic jam or other filling (see sidebar). Place the cookies on the baking sheet about 1 inch apart. Bake for about 15 minutes; the cookies are done when the bottoms are browned.

Makes 24 cookies

PER SERVING Calories: 132; Total Fat: 8 g (0 g saturated, 6 g monounsaturated); Carbohydrates: 14 g; Protein: 2 g; Fiber: 1 g; Sodium: 26 mg

INNER COOK NOTES

The choices of fillings are unlimited. Try organic almond or peanut butter (high in nutrients) topped with a few organic chocolate chips (omit the cinnamon, ginger, cardamom, and nutmeg for a more traditional cookie). Bake the cookies with chocolate chips and then sprinkle with toasted coconut when removed from the oven, or bake the cookies topped with raspberry jam and chocolate chips. You can also add $1/4$ cup currants or chopped raisins when you add the liquid. These cookies can be frozen in airtight containers for up to 1 month. Bring them to room temperature and warm for a few minutes in a 200°F oven.

Sometimes the toughest thing for someone recovering from cancer is ensuring their family eats well. The problem is compounded when little ones are involved. One woman recovering from colon cancer found this recipe to be family friendly. "My husband and I enjoy them, and we don't feel guilty eating them." She says her four-year-old helps, using her thumb to indent the cookie dough so they can be filled with peanut butter.

Flourless Almond Torte

IINNER COOK NOTES

This dessert is like a blank canvas . . . plenty of room for improvisation. During the summer, top the torte with blueberries, blackberries, or peaches; in the spring, top with fresh strawberries. In the fall, sauté apples and pears with a little bit of cinnamon, lemon juice, and a tablespoon of water; and in the winter, try adding 1 tablespoon orange zest to the batter and top your torte with ¼ cup of toasted coconut and 2 tablespoons of shaved dark chocolate. Yum! You could also try adding 1 tablespoon orange or lemon zest and currants, raisins, or dried cranberries to the batter. Or bake mini almond muffins with ¼ cup blueberries added to the batter.

Not all almond meal is created equal. Some brands of almond meal are coarsely ground, which gives the torte a rustic texture. If you want a smoother texture, or if you want to make your own almond meal, pulse 7 ounces of almonds until they are fine, but don't let them get oily. When they start to adhere to the side of the bowl, it's time to stop pulsing.

Even for the chronically baking-impaired, this is one of those easy desserts people will think you slaved over. This flourless torte relies on egg power for leavening, so beat those yolks until thick and foamy, but watch the egg whites—without added sugar they can get too dry in a hurry. Don't have a stand mixer? No problem! Pull out the hand mixer and whip yourself into a frenzy. If you beat the egg whites first, you won't have to wash the beaters when you move on to the yolks.

3 large organic eggs, at room temperature, separated (no yolk in the egg whites)	1 teaspoon almond extract
	2 cups (7 ounces) almond meal
¼ teaspoon sea salt	½ teaspoon vanilla extract
Pinch of cream of tartar (optional)	
⅓ cup maple syrup	Fresh seasonal fruit, for topping (optional)

Preheat the oven to 350°F. Line an 8-inch cake pan with a parchment paper circle cut to fit the bottom. Spray the sides lightly with natural oil spray.

Using a stand mixer fitted with the whisk, beat the egg whites with the salt and cream of tartar on medium high until stiff, but not dry, peaks form. Transfer the egg whites to a clean bowl.

Using the same mixer bowl (no need to wash bowl or whisk), add the yolks and beat on medium speed. Gradually add the maple syrup and the almond extract and beat on high speed until the mixture is thick, light in color, and foamy, about 4 to 5 minutes. Beat in the almond meal and the vanilla extract.

Fold the beaten egg whites into the batter quickly and gently with a rubber spatula, beginning by scooping in about one-fourth of the egg white mixture to lighten the batter. Fold in the remaining egg whites, taking care not to deflate the mixture too much.

Pour the batter into the prepared pan and smooth the top gently with a spatula. Bake for about 35 minutes, or until lightly browned and a toothpick inserted in the center comes out clean. Cool on a rack for 10 minutes. Run a small metal spatula around the edge of the pan and unmold the torte onto a lightly oiled rack. Reinvert the cake to cool completely.

Serve in wedges, topped with your favorite seasonal fruit.

Serves 8

PER SERVING Calories: 200; Total Fat: 14 g (1 g saturated, 8 g monounsaturated); Carbohydrates: 14 g; Protein: 7 g; Fiber: 3 g; Sodium: 101 mg

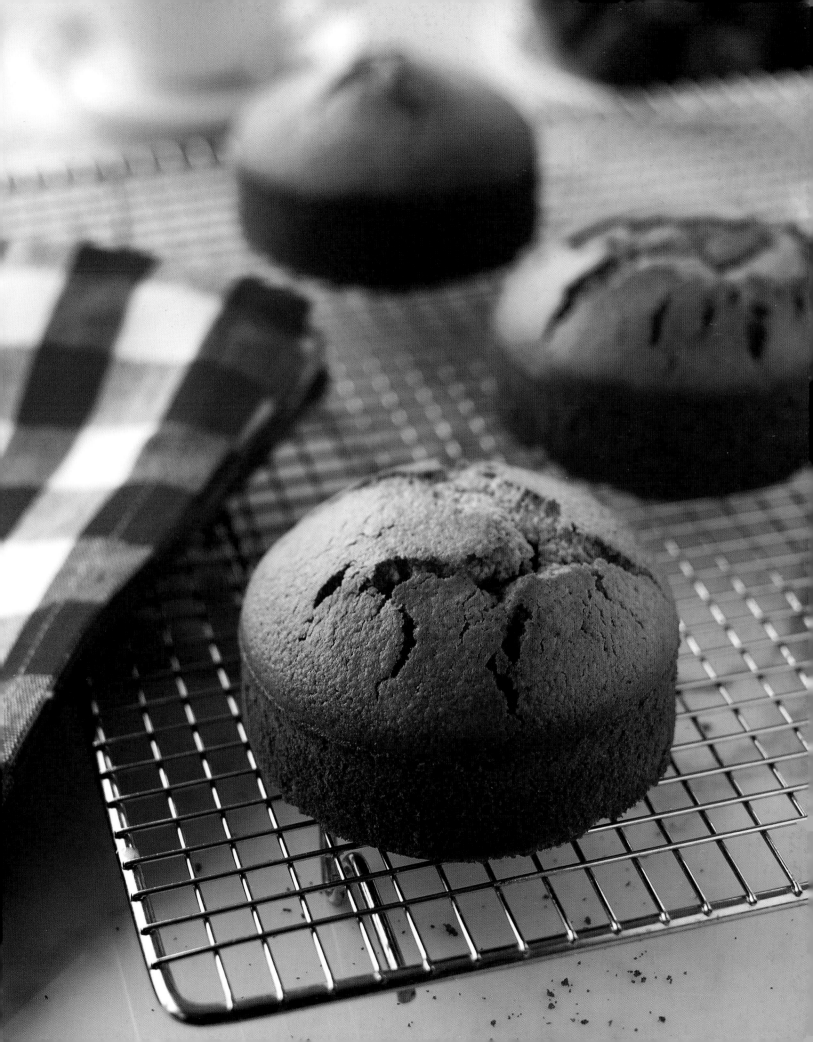

Chocolate-Orange Spice Muffins

My friend, a breast cancer survivor who's always eating on the go, loves to pour the Flourless Almond Torte batter into a mini-muffin tin and bake muffins to carry around in the car for a high-protein snack. I took her idea a little further and added cocoa and orange zest to make these tasty little muffins.

Zest of 1 orange, grated

3 tablespoons sifted cocoa powder

1 teaspoon ground cinnamon

$1/2$ teaspoon ground allspice

$1/4$ teaspoon ground cardamom

Freshly grated nutmeg

2 cups (7 ounces) almond meal

3 large organic eggs, at room temperature, separated (no yolk in the egg whites)

$1/4$ teaspoon sea salt

Pinch of cream of tartar (optional)

$1/3$ cup plus 1 tablespoon maple syrup

$1/4$ teaspoon vanilla extract

Preheat the oven to 350°F.

Add the orange zest, cocoa powder, cinnamon, allspice, cardamom, and a few gratings of nutmeg to the almond meal. Use your fingers to mix, breaking up any clumps.

Using a stand mixer fitted with the whisk, beat the egg whites with the salt and cream of tartar on medium high until stiff, but not dry, peaks form. Transfer the egg whites to a clean bowl.

Using the same mixer bowl (no need to wash bowl or whisk), add the yolks and beat on medium speed. Gradually add the maple syrup and beat on high speed until the mixture is thick, light in color, and foamy, about 4 to 5 minutes. Beat in the almond meal mixture and the vanilla extract.

Fold the beaten egg whites into the batter quickly and gently with a rubber spatula, beginning by scooping in about one-fourth of the egg white mixture to lighten the batter. Fold in the remaining egg whites, taking care not to deflate the mixture too much.

Scoop the batter into a muffin tin lined with muffin cups, filling each cup almost to the top. Bake for 12 to 15 minutes. Cool on a rack for 10 minutes, then remove the muffins from the pan and cool completely.

Serves 8

PER SERVING Calories: 218; Total Fat: 14 g (1 g saturated, 8 g monounsaturated); Carbohydrates: 17 g; Protein: 7 g; Fiber: 3 g; Sodium: 101 mg

Gingerbread

When I was growing up my mom made the most incredible gingerbread, which we smothered in applesauce. One day our recipe tester Linda and I were making soup for about a dozen students when it suddenly hit me. "I wish we had some gingerbread to go with this," I said. "I have a great recipe for gingerbread," replied Linda. She did. Using maple crystals, which result from exaporating granulated maple syrup, greatly cuts the sugar load without sacrificing any taste. This goes from the mixing bowl to pan to oven to plate to mouth in less than an hour. It makes the house smell delightful, too.

$1^2/_3$ cups organic, unbleached all-purpose flour or spelt, plus extra for dusting

$1^1/_4$ teaspoons baking soda

1 teaspoon ground ginger

$1/_2$ teaspoon ground cinnamon

$3/_4$ teaspoon sea salt

1 teaspoon grated fresh ginger

1 large organic egg

$1/_2$ cup maple crystals

$1/_2$ cup unsulfured blackstrap molasses

$1/_2$ cup boiling water

$1/_2$ cup safflower oil, plus extra for coating the pan

Preheat the oven to 350°F. Lightly oil and flour a 9-inch square baking dish or 2 small loaf pans.

Sift the flour, baking soda, ground ginger, cinnamon, salt, and fresh ginger into a bowl.

In a separate bowl, whisk together the egg, maple crystals, and molasses. Pour into the dry ingredients (the mixture will look like thick cookie dough at this point).

Pour the boiling water and the $1/_2$ cup oil over the batter and mix thoroughly with an electric mixer until smooth.

Pour the batter into the prepared pan(s). Bake on the middle rack of the oven for 35 to 40 minutes, or until the edges have slightly pulled away from the pan. Transfer from the oven to a cooling rack. Cool to room temperature in the pan. Transfer from the pan, slice, and serve on a platter.

Makes 1 (9-inch) square loaf or 2 small loaves (Serves 12)

PER SERVING Calories: 207; Total Fat: 10 g (0 g saturated, 8 g monounsaturated); Carbohydrates: 28 g; Protein: 2 g; Fiber: 0 g; Sodium: 186 mg

IINNER COOK NOTES
To lightly oil the pan, use a paper towel with a small amount of safflower oil. You can dust the pan with cocoa powder instead of flour.

I have made this recipe in a food processor as follows: Put the dry ingredients in and pulse for 30 seconds. Add the fresh ginger, maple crystals, egg, and molasses and process for 1 minute. Pour the water and oil through the feed tube and process until thoroughly mixed. Pour into the baking pan(s) and bake as directed.

Fruit Parfait with Almond-Peach-Ginger Cream

FRUIT PARFAIT

1 tablespoon kudzu root powder

2 1/2 cups chilled unsweetened apple juice

2 tablespoons agar agar flakes

2 cups chopped fresh fruit

ALMOND-PEACH-GINGER CREAM

1 cup raw blanched almonds

1 teaspoon fresh lemon juice

1/4 teaspoon sea salt

2 tablespoons maple syrup

1/4 teaspoon almond extract

1/2 teaspoon vanilla extract

1 teaspoon grated fresh ginger, or 1/2 teaspoon powdered ginger

Pinch of ground cinnamon

1/8 teaspoon freshly grated nutmeg

2 medium ripe peaches, peeled, pitted, and sliced

To make the fruit parfait, in a small bowl, add the kudzu to 1/2 cup of the apple juice. Whisk to dissolve and set aside.

In a medium pot, combine the remaining 2 cups apple juice, the agar agar, and half the fruit. Bring to a boil over high heat, decrease the heat to low, and simmer for about 5 minutes, or until the agar agar is thoroughly dissolved.

Whisk the kudzu mixture into the hot liquid, stirring constantly, until the mixture just starts to bubble again. Immediately remove from the heat, pour into a heat-resistant shallow pan, cool to room temperature, and refrigerate until firmly set.

To make the almond cream, pour 1 cup water into a blender or your Vita-Mix followed by the almonds, lemon juice, salt, maple syrup, extracts, ginger, cinnamon, nutmeg, and peaches. Blend until very, very smooth. Add a squeeze of lemon juice or a pinch of salt to finish, if necessary.

Transfer the parfait from the refrigerator to a food processor fitted with a metal blade and process until smooth. Pour into a medium bowl and fold in the second cup of fruit. Pour into a clear glass bowl, or individual serving bowls in alternating layers with the Almond-Peach-Ginger Cream. Chill and serve.

Serves 8

PER SERVING Calories: 148; Total Fat: 6 g (0 g saturated, 4 g monounsaturated); Carbohydrates: 22 g; Protein: 3 g; Fiber: 2 g; Sodium: 85 g

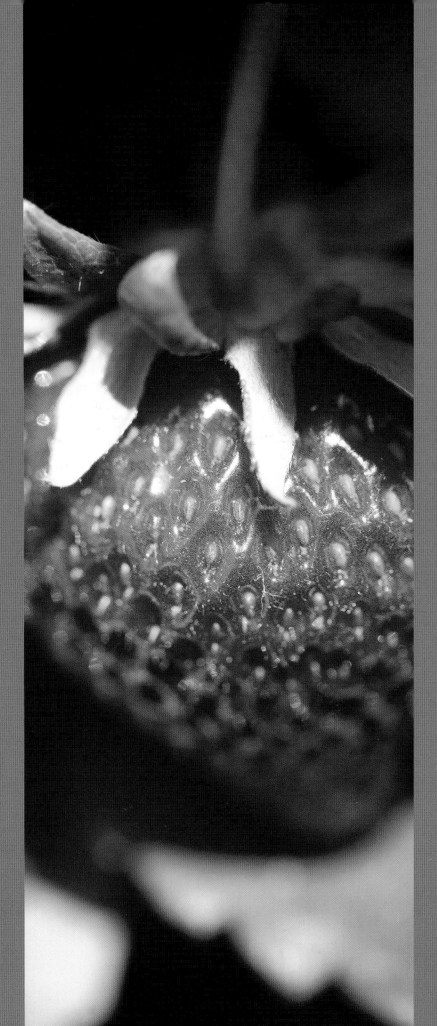

Chapter 8 Dollops of Yum

Like a lovely ribbon around a beautiful present, I'm always looking for ways to surround my recipes with something extraordinary, a special sauce or dressing that is absolutely fabulous. Welcome to dollops of yum!

REMEMBER LICKING THE FROSTING OFF THE SPOON WHEN YOU WERE A KID? That's the same feeling these dollops evoke. Pistachio Mint Pesto (page 25). Lemon Cashew Cream (page 119). Grandma Nora's Salsa Verde (page 117). Alone, they're incredible. Put them over greens, fish, chicken, or veggies and you'll be able to plead temporary insanity.

The difference with these dollops is they're actually good for you. Immunity builders. That's not true of most commercial salad dressings and dips. That's why the recipes in this chapter are mostly made with lemons, limes, and oranges instead of vinegar: These fruits are higher in healthy phytochemicals and, just as important, they have a fresher taste!

These dollops are extremely versatile and act as the perfect accompaniment to jazz up light fare such as pita or toast. Of course, you could just lick these straight off a spoon. I promise I won't tell.

Avocado Cream

Somewhere, somehow, avocados got a bad rap. Yes, they're high in fat, but it's good monounsaturated fat. They're also loaded with vitamin B₆, potassium, and a host of other nutrients. The only other fruit that comes close to this nutritional profile is an olive. Between the olive oil and avocado, this has to be the healthiest cream on the planet. Might be the tastiest, too. This is great spread on sandwiches or dolloped on dishes throughout this book.

1 ripe avocado, coarsley chopped	**1 tablespoon water**
¹/₄ cup loosely packed fresh cilantro (optional)	**1 tablespoon fresh lime juice**
	¹/₄ teaspoon sea salt

In a blender or a food processor fitted with a metal blade, combine the avocado, cilantro, water, lime juice, and salt and process until smooth. Think FASS: You may want to add some extra lime juice or a pinch of salt.

Makes 1 cup

PER SERVING (1 tablespoon per serving) Calories: 20; Total Fat: 2 g (0 g saturated, 1 g monounsaturated); Carbohydrates: 1 g; Protein: 0 g; Fiber: 1 g; Sodium: 38 mg

INNER COOK NOTES
Want a little heat? Add a pinch of cayenne.

Sometimes I want this cream so badly that I invent ways to have it. Once I sliced jicama into matchsticks to dip into it rather than chips. It was great!

Basil and Arugula Pesto

1 cup chopped baby arugula, stems removed	**1¹/₂ tablespoons fresh lemon juice**
¹/₄ cup fresh basil leaves	**¹/₄ teaspoon maple syrup**
¹/₄ teaspoon minced garlic	**¹/₄ teaspoon sea salt**
	¹/₄ cup extra virgin olive oil

Place the arugula, basil, garlic, lemon juice, maple syrup, and salt in a food processor fitted with a metal blade. Process until finely chopped. While the processor is running, slowly drizzle the olive oil through the feed tube and continue to process until very smooth.

Taste and think about FASS. Arugula, fresh herbs, and lemons can vary in the intensity of their flavor; for example, arugula may be bitter and the lemons tart, so you may need to add more basil, a few drops of olive oil or maple syrup, or another pinch of salt.

Makes ¹/₂ cup

PER SERVING (1 tablespoon per serving) Calories: 63; Total Fat: 7g (1 g saturated, 5 g monounsaturated); Carbohydrates: 1 g; Protein: 0 g; Fiber: 0 g; Sodium: 74 mg

INNER COOK NOTES
If you want a richer or thicker sauce, add a handful of pistachios or pine nuts to the food processor. The nuts will add more depth to the flavor and make the sauce perfect for spreading on a sandwich or crostini.

Fruit Compote

This is a superb recipe for people on pain medication. Such medications can be extremely binding. This compote—how can I put this gently?—keeps the backfield in motion. The compote is made with dried fruit such as prunes, apricots, and raisins. They're simmered for a while on the stove top and infused with cardamom and ginger for depth and to aid in digestion. This compote is outstanding spread on toast or dolloped on oatmeal.

INNER COOK NOTES
You can use dried apples, pears, figs, or any combination of dried fruit to equal 3 cups.

This dish smells incredible while it's cooking. It keeps in the refrigerator for up to a week and can be frozen in small airtight containers for up to 3 months.

The compote is a versatile condiment that crosses culinary boundaries and can be used in both sweet and savory dishes. Put it on yogurt, a sweet potato, or the Best Oatmeal Ever (page 84). You can even eat a dollop spread on a piece of toast.

1 cup pitted prunes

1 cup unsulfured dried apricots

1 cup dried cherries or raisins

3 cinnamon sticks

6 cardamom pods, or $1/4$ teaspoon ground cardamom

$1/2$ teaspoon chopped fresh ginger, or $1/4$ teaspoon powdered ginger

Pinch of sea salt

$1/4$ teaspoon fresh lemon juice

Place the prunes, apricots, cherries, cinnamon, cardamom, ginger, and salt in a medium saucepan. Add water to cover the fruit. Soak overnight, if possible, or for a few hours before cooking.

Bring the mixture to a boil over high heat. Decrease the heat to low and slowly simmer for about 1 hour, or until all the ingredients are very, very soft and the liquid has become syrupy. Stir in the lemon juice.

Makes 4 to 5 cups

PER SERVING Calories: 75; Total Fat: 0 g (0 g saturated, 0 g monounsaturated); Carbohydrates: 18 g; Protein: 1 g; Fiber: 3 g; Sodium: 16 mg

Pistachio Cream

1 cup water

2 teaspoons fresh lemon juice

$1/4$ teaspoon sea salt

1 cup shelled raw pistachios

In a blender, combine the water, lemon juice, salt, and pistachios. Blend until very smooth.

Makes $1^1/2$ cups

PER SERVING Calories: 30; Total Fat: 2 g (0 g saturated, 1 g monounsaturated); Carbohydrates: 1 g; Protein: 1 g; Fiber: 0 g; Sodium: 25 mg

Grandma Nora's Salsa Verde

Grandma Nora was pretty wild. She looked more like Sophia Loren than a typical Italian nonna and held court at a sixteenth-century villa in Palermo. She also preferred cooking with a glass of homemade red wine in one hand and a spoon in the other. She taught me this simple, fresh, and tasty sauce. The anchovies are barely discernible but add a nice boost of omega-3 fatty acids. This sauce is so flavorful that we used to sit around the villa and dunk bread in it. The parsley alone is full of oxygen. It's like eating fresh air all year round.

2 bunches fresh flat-leaf parsley (about 2 cups)

$^1/_4$ cup extra virgin olive oil

2 anchovies (optional)

2 cloves garlic, finely chopped

1 tablespoon fresh lemon juice

Pinch of sea salt

Rinse the parsley and shake off any excess water. Remove the stems (see Parsley "Haircut" on page 151, for a fast, easy method). Process the parsley in a food processor fitted with a metal blade for about 30 seconds, scraping down the sides afterward.

Add the olive oil, anchovies, garlic, lemon juice, and salt. Process until smooth, stopping and scraping down the sides a couple of times.

Think FASS: You may need to add another pinch of salt or a few more drops of olive oil.

Makes about $^1/_2$ cup

PER SERVING (1 tablespoon per serving) Calories: 67; Total Fat: 7 g (1 g saturated, 5 g mono-unsaturated); Carbohydrates: 1 g; Protein: 1 g; Fiber: 1 g; Sodium: 27 mg

INNER COOK NOTES

If you want a richer or thicker salsa, add a handful of pistachios to the food processor. The nuts will add more depth to the flavor and make the sauce perfect for spreading on a sandwich or a crostini.

If you want a thinner salsa verde, add 1 tablespoon of water and process until you reach the desired consistency.

Skip the anchovies if you don't like them; the sauce is still outstanding. In the summertime, add fresh basil or mint to the mix for extra pizzazz. Drizzle on meat, chicken, or vegetables. Toss with pasta or drizzle on soups or polenta. Do your salmon or favor-ite fish a favor and drench them with this. They'll give you the thumbs up.

Herbed "Ricotta"

INNER COOK NOTES
Try this as a spread on crostini, or as the first layer on your cornmeal crust pizza. We also use this in Veggie "Ricotta" Lasagna (page 77). If you like galettes, try spreading this on the bottom of the galettes and filling them with Delicata Squash with Dino Kale and Cranberries (page 41).

Let's face it: Most tofu resembles a pair of old sneakers in both rubbery texture and taste. That's a shame because properly prepared tofu is delightful. Tofu is the chameleon of the bean world in that it completely takes on surrounding flavors. As for texture, all tofu needs to become smooth and creamy is to have a little up-close and personal time with a food processor. The addition of miso gives this tofu a cheeselike sensibility, while the other herbs and spices punch up the taste.

1 pound firm tofu, quartered, rinsed, drained, and patted dry

1 tablespoon white miso

2 teaspoons fresh lemon juice

$1/2$ teaspoon sea salt

1 teaspoon crushed fennel seeds

1 teaspoon freshly grated nutmeg

$1/8$ teaspoon ground cinnamon

1 teaspoon lemon zest

$1/4$ cup extra virgin olive oil

1 teaspoon chopped fresh oregano

1 tablespoon finely chopped fresh flat-leaf parsley

1 tablespoon chopped fresh basil

Crumble the tofu into the bowl of a food processor fitted with a metal blade and process for 1 minute. Add the miso, lemon juice, salt, fennel seeds, nutmeg, cinnamon, and lemon zest and pulse to combine.

With the processor running, slowly add the olive oil and continue processing until the mixture is smooth and creamy. Scrape down the sides and process for another 30 seconds. Taste at this point; you're looking for a velvety texture. If it's not velvety smooth, add some additional olive oil, $1/4$ teaspoon at a time, process, and taste again.

When the mixture is velvety smooth, add the oregano, parsley, and basil, process, and taste again. Think FASS: You may need a squeeze of lemon juice or a pinch of salt.

Makes 2 cups

PER SERVING Calories: 121; Total Fat: 7 g (1 g saturated, 5 g monounsaturated); Carbohydrates: 2 g; Protein: 7 g; Fiber: 1 g; Sodium: 200 mg

Lemon Cashew Cream

Folks often assume you have to use butter to get a buttery taste, but crushed cashews yield a similar flavor. It's a top-notch alternative for those who want to limit their dairy intake. I create this cream using either lemon juice and water or Magic Mineral Broth (page 13). Purée it in a blender until it's very creamy.

2 cups raw cashews

2 cups water

2 teaspoons fresh lemon juice

$1/2$ teaspoon sea salt

$1/8$ to $1/4$ teaspoon freshly grated nutmeg

Grind the cashews in a mini food processor or nut grinder to give them a head start in the blender. Most blenders can't go from nuts to cream without a jump start. If you have a Vita-Mix, you can skip this step. Put 2 cups of water in your blender. Add the lemon juice, salt, nutmeg, and cashews. Blend until creamy smooooooooth; be patient (this takes several minutes). Your patience will be rewarded when your taste buds are covered in cashmere.

Makes about $3^1/2$ cups

PER SERVING (1 tablespoon per serving) Calories: 29; Total Fat: 2 g (0 g saturated, 1 g mono-unsaturated); Carbohydrates: 2 g; Protein: 1 g; Fiber: 0 g; Sodium: 22 mg

INNER COOK NOTES
Variations: Substitute other nuts, such as almonds, pecans, pistachio, or hazelnuts, or add $1^1/2$ cups fresh basil and toss with your favorite pasta or rice.

Use it to top soups and veggies or toss it with orzo for a dairy-free "mac and cheese."

Lemon Caper Vinaigrette

We call it the "waker-upper" dressing! It has bright lively flavors that wake up your taste buds. This dressing swings both ways! It's a salad dressing or a great marinade for chicken or fish. Make a batch at the last minute or ahead of time.

$1/4$ cup fresh lemon juice

$1/2$ teaspoon organic honey

1 teaspoon minced garlic

1 teaspoon minced shallot

$1/4$ teaspoon Dijon mustard

1 tablespoon capers, rinsed

Pinch of sea salt

Pinch of freshly ground pepper

$1/4$ cup extra virgin olive oil

In a small mixing bowl, whisk together the lemon juice, honey, garlic, shallot, and mustard. Add the capers, salt, and pepper. Slowly whisk in the olive oil. Dip in a lettuce leaf and taste the dressing. You may want to add another pinch of salt.

Makes about 1 cup

PER SERVING (1 tablespoon per serving) Calories: 33; Total Fat: 4 g (0 g saturated, 3 g mono-unsaturated); Carbohydrates: 1 gram; Protein: 0 g; Fiber: 0 g; Sodium: 27 mg

INNER COOK NOTES
The dressing will keep for up to 1 week in the refrigerator.

Puttanesca Sauce

Some people asked me why I was putting a spicy puttanesca sauce into this book. I've found that the saltiness of the capers and olives is appealing to those with compromised taste buds, and a little kick from the red pepper flakes seals the deal. This sauce is excellent over pasta, fish, and chicken and on pizza and creamy polenta.

INNER COOK NOTES
A 26-ounce can of whole tomatoes can be used in place of fresh Roma tomatoes. To roast canned tomatoes, spread them on a sheet pan, sprinkle with ½ teaspoon rapadura, and drizzle with olive oil. Roast for 6 to 8 minutes, remove from the oven, and set aside until ready to use.

Puttenesca is traditionally made with anchovies, but not everyone likes their taste. If that's the case, drop the fish and you've still got a scrumptious sauce. If you want a plain tomato sauce, skip the olives, capers, and red pepper flakes. Roast the tomatoes and add chopped fresh basil.

The Big O: Using conventionally grown tomatoes in a sauce is like building a home on quicksand. Good luck getting such mealy, tasteless, watered-downed tomatoes to stand-up to any discerning palate! In my opinion, organic tomatoes win hands-down on taste, flavor, texture, and juiciness. As for nutrition, the U.S. Department of Agriculture found organic tomatoes have higher natural levels of the antioxidant lycopene, and cooking these tomatoes pushes those levels to even greater heights.

2 pounds Roma tomatoes, halved, or 1 (26-ounce) can of whole tomatoes with the juice

3 tablespoons extra virgin olive oil

1 teaspoon rapadura or other organic sweetener

¼ teaspoon sea salt

2 teaspoons minced garlic

Pinch of red pepper flakes

¼ cup dry white wine or water

½ cup sliced pitted black olives (Gaeta or kalamata)

1½ tablespoons capers, rinsed and chopped

2 anchovy fillets, rinsed and chopped (optional)

1 teaspoon chopped fresh flat-leaf parsley, or ½ teaspoon chopped fresh mint, for garnish

Preheat the oven to 400°F.

Toss the tomatoes with 2 tablespoons of the olive oil, the rapadura, and salt. Place cut side down on a sheet pan with sides. Roast for 15 to 20 minutes, or until golden and bubbly. Transfer the tomatoes with a slotted spoon to your food processor and pulse several times; the tomatoes should remain chunky.

In a heavy sauté pan over medium-high heat, heat the remaining 1 tablespoon olive oil. Add the garlic and red pepper flakes and cook for 30 seconds, until just aromatic. Add the wine and simmer for about 1 minute. Add the tomatoes and simmer until the sauce is slightly thickened, 5 to 10 minutes. Stir in the olives, capers, and anchovies.

Taste: Think FASS. You may need a pinch of sweetener to round out the flavor. Garnish with the parsley before serving.

Makes about 2 cups (Serves 4)

PER SERVING Calories: 230; Total Fat: 15 g (2 g saturated, 11 g monounsaturated); Carbohydrates: 17 g; Protein: 3 g; Fiber: 4 g; Sodium: 585 mg

Blueprint for Yummy Salsas

In Louisiana they would call this the two-step Mamou; it's fun no matter which foot you put forward. Salsa Cruda (below), which blends fresh tomatoes and spices, is super on vegetables and eggs, but I've found fish and poultry lovers prefer a sweeter taste, which is where the fruit salsa (page 122) takes the floor. I whirl luscious mangoes and papayas in the mix, but pineapple can also step in. Sometimes you just want a great dance partner. Or two.

2 cups chopped pineapple, papaya, mango, avocado, or a combination

Red bell pepper or jalapeño peppers, seeded and finely chopped

Fresh herbs, such as cilantro, flat-leaf parsley, chives, and mint, coarsely chopped

Sweet red onion

Extra virgin olive oil

Fresh lime or lemon juice

Sea salt

Mix all the ingredients in a bowl and let stand for 30 minutes to allow the flavors to mingle. The salsa is best eaten the day it's prepared, but it will hold in the refrigerator, tightly covered, for several days. After a few days, the flavor may fade a bit, so add a few drops of lemon or lime juice to freshen it up.

Makes about 2 cups

Salsa Cruda

1¹/₂ cups diced Roma tomatoes

¹/₄ cup diced red onion

2 tablespoons chopped fresh cilantro

1 to 2 teaspoons fresh lime juice

1 teaspoon seeded, ribbed, and diced jalapeño

¹/₄ teaspoon sea salt

In a medium bowl, mix all the ingredients together. Taste and adjust the flavors. Let the salsa sit for 30 minutes and taste again. Bump up the jalapeño for some heat!

Makes about 2 cups

PER SERVING Calories: 8; Total Fat: 0 g (0 g saturated, 0 g monounsaturated); Carbohydrates: 2 g; Protein: 0 g; Fiber: 0 g; Sodium: 78 mg

Fruit and Fresh Herb Salsa

INNER COOK NOTES
Substitute fennel or radishes for the red bell pepper for a twist.

2 ripe mangoes, peeled and diced, or 1 ripe pineapple (or a combination), to make 2 cups of chopped fruit

3 tablespoons finely diced red bell pepper

3 tablespoons finely chopped fresh cilantro

1 tablespoon finely chopped fresh mint

1 teaspoon seeded and finely diced jalapeño, or a generous pinch of cayenne

1 tablespoon extra virgin olive oil

2 tablespoons fresh lime juice

$1/4$ teaspoon sea salt

In a medium bowl, mix all the ingredients together. Taste and think FASS. Let the salsa sit for 30 minutes, taste again, and dollop on your favorite food or serve as a dip for pita crisps or jicama sticks.

Makes about $2^1/_2$ cups

PER SERVING (2 tablespoons per serving) Calories: 28; Total Fat: 0 g (0 g saturated, 0 g mono-unsaturated); Carbohydrates: 7 g; Protein: 0 g; Fiber: 1 g; Sodium: 62 mg

Sea-ser Dressing

INNER COOK NOTES
Purée in your food processor or blender for a creamier texture. Store the extra in the refrigerator for up to a week.

A lot of people avoid eating sea vegetables because they've never been exposed to them before. That's a shame, because these vegetables have outstanding detoxifying properties. This dressing is a super way to agreeably introduce folks to sea veggies. As one of my clients said: "It was the best Caesar dressing I've ever tasted. It was very well-appointed."

No, that's not a misspelling: This is a twist on conventional Caesar dressing. Out go the anchovies, replaced by dulse flakes. Never heard of dulse? It's a nutrient-rich sea vegetable that does a lovely imitation of those teeny-tiny fish. Toss this dressing on top of romaine or mixed greens and challenge your friends to tell you what's different about the dressing.

2 teaspoons Dijon mustard

$1/4$ cup fresh lime juice

$1^1/_2$ teaspoons dulse flakes

$1/2$ teaspoon Worcestershire sauce or vegetarian Worcestershire sauce

2 cloves garlic, minced

$1/4$ teaspoon sea salt

$1/2$ cup extra virgin olive oil

Mix the mustard, lime juice, dulse flakes, Worcestershire sauce, garlic, salt, and $1/4$ cup water in a small bowl. Slowly add the olive oil in a steady stream, whisking constantly until emulsified.

Makes about 1 cup

PER SERVING (1 tablespoon per serving) Calories: 62; Total Fat: 7 g (1 g saturated, 5 g mono-unsaturated); Carbohydrates: 0 g; Protein: 0 g; Fiber: 0 g; Sodium: 47 mg

Sweet "Ricotta"

As with the Herbed "Ricotta" (page 118), you'll have a hard time believing this isn't cheese, but tofu. This sweet citrus "ricotta" uses orange juice, orange zest, a tad of Grade B organic maple syrup, and some warming spices. Add a shaving of nutmeg and you have an ideal filling for the Cashew Tart Crust (page 106).

1 pound firm tofu, quartered, rinsed, drained, and patted dry	$1^1/_2$ teaspoons freshly grated nutmeg
1 tablespoon white miso	$1/_8$ teaspoon ground cinnamon
$1/_4$ cup fresh lemon juice	1 tablespoon powdered ginger
3 tablespoons fresh orange juice	1 tablespoon grated orange zest
1 teaspoon sea salt	1 tablespoon grated lemon zest
$1/_4$ cup maple syrup	$1/_4$ cup extra virgin olive oil

Crumble the tofu into the bowl of a food processor fitted with a metal blade and pulse for 1 minute.

Add the miso, lemon and orange juices, salt, maple syrup, nutmeg, cinnamon, ginger, and orange and lemon zests and pulse for another minute.

With the processor running, slowly add the olive oil through the feed tube and process until the mixture is smooth and very creamy.

Taste and think FASS: You may need to add another squeeze of lemon or orange juice, or a drop of maple syrup.

Serves 8

PER SERVING Calories: 157; Total Fat: 11 g (2 g saturated, 5 g monounsaturated); Carbohydrates: 10 g; Protein: 7 g; Fiber: 1 g; Sodium: 361 mg

Keeping up culinary rituals is one way of staying grounded during and after cancer treatment. One woman loved eating fruit and cheese in the evening with her husband, but her practitioner suggested she give up dairy for a month as one way to clean out her system. This recipe allowed her to continue her nightly dessert sessions with her spouse. The faux ricotta was so sweet, she took to dipping strawberries in it. The first time she tried this, she turned to me and said "Oh, my . . . . Aaaaah! This is a great trick. That's a solution!"

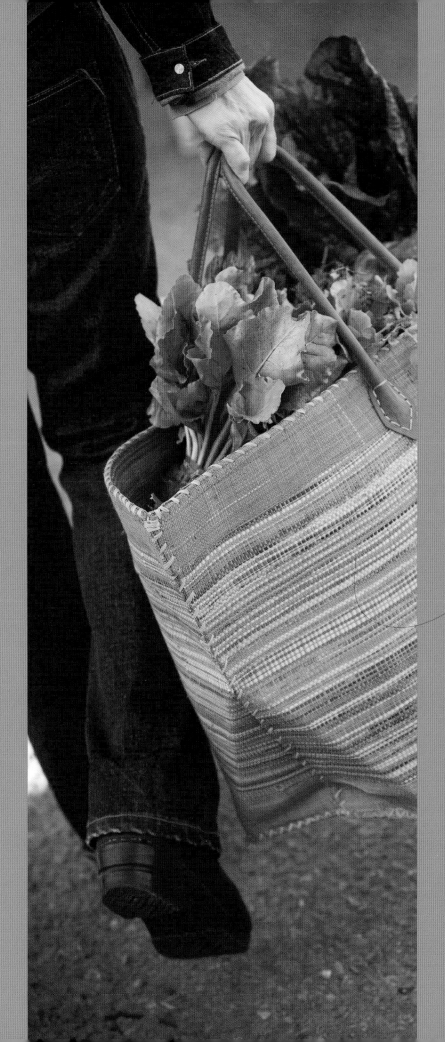

Sharing a delicious meal we could all enjoy made me feel like a normal person. I could sit down and eat with everyone. Then there's the conversation at mealtime. I didn't feel isolated. A lot of days I couldn't go out, so people would come to me. It always helped.

—Shannon McGowan, lung cancer survivor

CAREGIVERS LITERALLY GIVE COMFORT, AID, AND SUSTENANCE TO A PERSON IN NEED. Taken to its highest level, caregiving defines a loving relationship: You *care* about the person you're supporting because you know they truly care about you. When we're talking about friends and family acting as caregivers, it's easy to assume that such a role comes naturally. Perhaps it does, but cancer has a way of throwing up emotional roadblocks that inhibit the caregiving process. Lowering those barriers, improving communication, and doing what needs to be done so that, from a culinary viewpoint, you're really caregiving. You've read Shannon's words above. Joining together over the table, sharing our days, and honoring each other's presence over a wonderful meal is always life affirming. These moments take on treasured poignancy (or just some much-needed normalcy!) when someone is going through cancer as a patient or a caregiver.

Whether you're a friend, family member, or concerned acquaintance, becoming an effective culinary caregiver means pushing past the emotions that inhibit you from reaching out. Fear, pride, guilt, embarrassment: anything that gets in the way of common sense and clear conversation needs to take a hike. Pick up the phone, send an email, hire a blimp to do a flyover, walk across the den, do whatever you have to do, but please let that special someone know that you want to bring them a bite to eat. If *you* are that special someone used to being the family caregiver, accepting help can be especially difficult. My suggestion is to see gestures of support as loving gifts and an opportunity to gently guide your caregivers in making you the foods you truly need.

Caregivers greatly benefit from such guidance. Cooking for someone with cancer isn't the same as cooking for someone who is healthy. Cancer and its treatments may wreak havoc on your friend's taste buds, digestion, and energy. One week they won't want to touch food, and the next week they'll eat like a linebacker. Sometimes there's no rhyme or reason to these appetite swings, which can prove frustrating to caregivers. It may be disappointing when you show up at the front door with their usual favorite meal and they look at it as if it were a platter of live octopi. If someone has had chemo within the last day or two, they probably can't handle your prize-winning Tuna Noodle Mexicali Bake. That's not to say they don't want nourishment—they do—but they are apt to want something far lighter, such as a few sips of warm tea or broth.

I've found the best way for caregivers to ride through a patient's highs and lows is to lower their expectations and stay flexible. Don't expect a patient to eat on a regular schedule. The concepts of breakfast, lunch, and dinner time no longer apply. Anytime a cancer patient wants to eat anything consider that great news, even if it's the same item for days on end. As for finishing off a dish, that's not going to happen when you cook for someone with cancer. At least not all the time. People with end-stage cancer may hardly be able to eat, yet many of them still want to enjoy food. A hospice nurse told me that some of her clients like to just nibble on tiny portions of their favorite foods. It may seem like a waste of time to cook for someone in this state. I assure you it's not.

When deciding what to cook, you must be flexible. This means making sure the person you're caring for has lots of different meals on hand, everything from extremely light fare (soups) to something more hearty (veggies, poultry, and the like). Most of the recipes in this book store well in the fridge or freezer in individual containers, ready to be reheated and served in a flash, with all of their delightful original flavors intact. My goal when I cook for someone dealing with cancer is pretty simple: no matter what they may want (outside of a Snickers bar), they'll be able to look in their freezer or fridge after I've gone and find something that satisfies.

Of course, that's a lot to ask from one caregiver. That's why I suggest that friends and family build a culinary support team *before* cancer treatment begins. That gives caregivers time to implement a plan and allows the word to get out to the community. The response may overwhelm you— it comes from all points on one's social, business, and family map—and everyone can contribute to ensuring that someone with cancer is well fed.

There are two good reasons to cast a wide net when putting together a culinary team. Such caregiving may go on for some time. Having a large support system means that no one gets burned out emotionally or physically. People can come and go as their schedule allows. Another reason to have a big team is to split up chores. Not everyone wants to be a cook. One family I know had a friend who kept them well stocked in paper goods from a local Costco. Another family included a sister who didn't cook but loved going to the farmers' market. Guess who did the shopping for them? Dividing the cooking chores, coming up with a designated chopper, finding a volunteer for dish washing

duties . . . it all goes more smoothly when everyone feels like they're part of a healing team.

Such a team does more than support; it allows someone who is sick to participate as little or as much as they want in the process. Shannon McGowan, whose comments led off this chapter, told me how much it meant to her to have friends come over and cook in her kitchen. It was a way for Shannon to judge her own recovery. Sometimes she could barely lift her head off the couch and watch. Then came the day when she wanted to do more. Though still weakened and barely able to walk, her friends knew what to do with Shannon. They led her into the kitchen, sat her down, and laid a small cutting board on her lap. On the board was fresh basil from her garden. Shannon's job—and it took every ounce of her strength—was to tightly roll and cut the basil as a garnish for braised artichokes. In that moment, in her kitchen, in her mind, Shannon was not a cancer patient; she was a cook whipping up a wonderful meal with—and for—her friends. At a time when so much was out of her control, this was something in her control, sharing something she cherishes with those who cherish her.

Two final thoughts for caregivers: The first is to take care of you, too. Caregiving is draining. The better you look after yourself, the more energy you'll have for others. The second thought especially pertains to people who don't cook, yet still want to be culinary caregivers. You can be simply by creating a pleasant environment for someone to enjoy a meal. So many cancer patients describe their life during chemo as flat, dull, and full of shades of gray. Want to make a difference in their life? Bring over fresh flowers, or a bright beautiful bowl they can eat soup in. See where I'm going here? Be creative; find those things that nourish your own soul and bring them to the kitchen of someone who is going through a tough time. You'll be amazed at how much healing power they have.

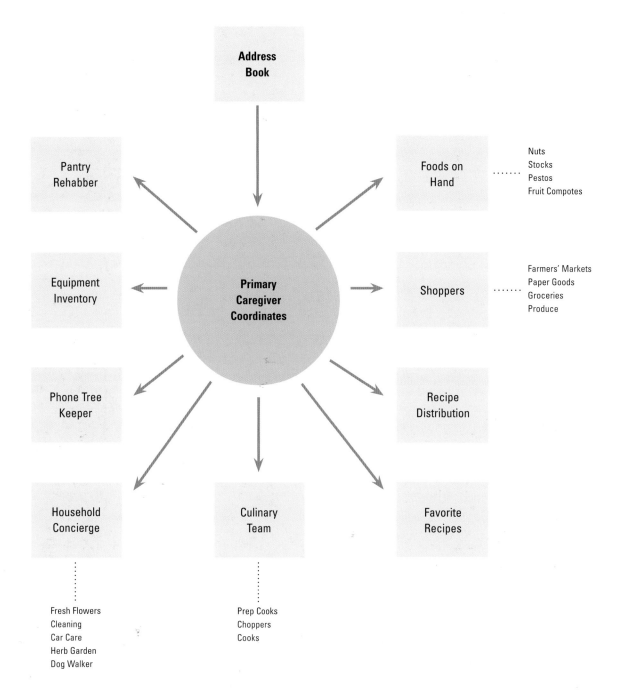

Address
Book

Pantry
Rehabber

Foods on
Hand

Nuts
Stocks
Pestos
Fruit Compotes

Equipment
Inventory

Primary
Caregiver
Coordinates

Shoppers

Farmers' Markets
Paper Goods
Groceries
Produce

Phone Tree
Keeper

Recipe
Distribution

Household
Concierge

Culinary
Team

Favorite
Recipes

Fresh Flowers
Cleaning
Car Care
Herb Garden
Dog Walker

Prep Cooks
Choppers
Cooks

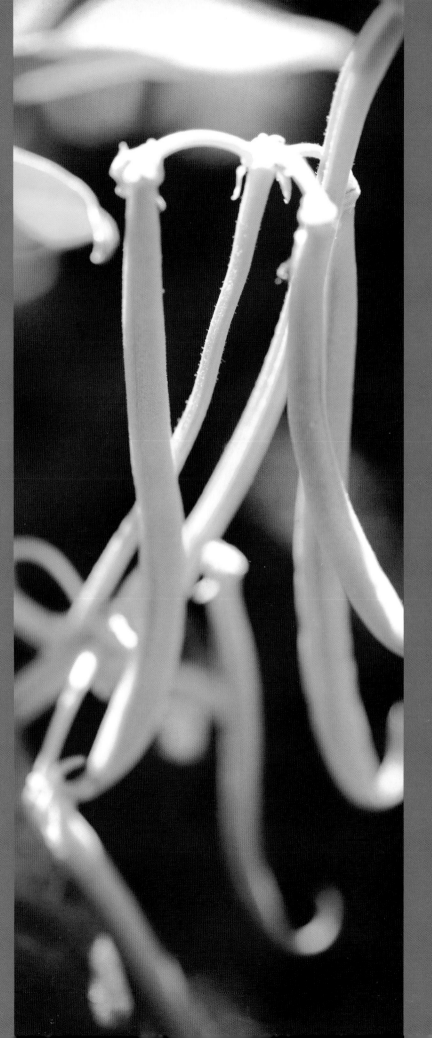

When people eat well, cook for themselves, their friends, and family, everything about their life slows down. It's like living in a small town. There's more communication together. It's like in those Frank Lloyd Wright homes: The kitchen is right in the middle. That's where everyone wants to be anyway.

—Michael Broffman, Director, Pine Street Clinic

IF YOU'RE READING THIS BOOK, CHANCES ARE YOU OR SOMEONE YOU LOVE IS IN A CRISIS. Hopefully that won't be the case for long. More people are beating cancer. Others, though not cancer free, are living longer with a better quality of life than they would have experienced a generation ago. That's great news. It also opens a doorway. I've found with my clients that going through a health crisis, while difficult, can have a galvanizing effect. They begin looking at ways to bring more joy into their lives. In other words, they want to learn how to nourish themselves.

Now, I'm not telling you whether you should quit your job and take off on a round-the-world trip or hike up the Himalayas (though both sound pretty good to me!). However, I do have some ideas that will help you reframe the way you approach food from here on out. I call it "sustainable nourishment." As the name suggests, the idea has several components. My friend, Michael Broffman, treats many people with cancer. Here in Marin County, California, we have one of the nation's highest breast cancer rates. Many patients come to Michael having been put on restricted diets by their physicians. Sometimes they've picked up information about what they should and should not be eating from their friends, television, or the Internet. The final effect is that they become extremely wary of food or, if they previously had food issues, those phobias now come to the fore. One of my clients, Aliyah, summed up this mind set.

"I became scared of food," she says. "I was so scared of eating anything bad for me that it was easier not to eat."

Most people can maintain a restricted diet for a short time, especially when they're first diagnosed. Over time, though, this can cause them to lose their connection to food. Whether you're healthy or sick, food is literally your connection to life. Sustainable nourishment is about making those connections within whatever framework is best for your health. It's also about realizing that there are often better-tasting and healthier alternatives to many of the foods you've grown accustomed to.

Linking healthy food with fabulous taste isn't an accident; it's a necessity. Even if the components of a food may be healthy, if it doesn't appeal to our taste buds, we're not likely to eat it. If we don't eat, we can't maintain our health.

So let's agree: Any food that's to be considered part of "sustainable nourishment" must titillate our taste buds. That's where the lessons learned in chapter 1 can help. But that's just a starting point. Although science is far from deciding whether certain foods cure cancer, evidence increasingly suggests that what we eat may help prevent cancer from initially occurring. Our first line of defense in battling illness is our immune system, and several food sources may boost its efficiency. These include antioxidants in vegetables and fruits, omega-3 fatty acids in some cold-water fish, and phytochemicals in plants. Such protection should be reason enough for anyone to gravitate toward these nourishing foods, especially those whose immune systems may have been affected by cancer treatments.

So now we have a fairly good working definition of sustainable nourishment. It involves food that both tastes great *and* contains the ingredients our body needs to sustain good health. So that rules out a steady cuisine of Twinkies (sorry). But I hope you realize by now that if you've looked at the recipes in this book, it doesn't rule out much else. My hope is that as you work your way through the book, new culinary possibilities will begin to percolate in your head. I'm looking for that epiphany, that "aha!" moment when you realize that healthy eating expands your options instead of restricting them. This is part of sustainable nourishment as well. Eating—and here I'm talking about sitting down to a nice meal, as opposed to doing the fast-food fandango—has positive psychological effects that translate into physiological results. Amazing things occur as one eats a satisfying, nourishing meal. Your heart rate and blood pressure decrease. Levels of cortisol, the hormone that surges when we're stressed, suddenly drop. Immunoglobulin levels, an indicator of the health of the immune system, begin to rise (that's good!). In fact, the satiation response is similar to what happens when people meditate.

In short, this kind of eating lowers the stressors that wear us out over time. That's why I think a huge part of sustainable nourishment also includes choosing and preparing one's own food. Many people I work with describe the mental zone they get into during cooking as being similar to the focused yet relaxed state achieved during meditation or yoga. Now that would be a fun comparison study to take part in!

It wouldn't surprise me if cooking provides physiological benefits. Whether or not that's ever been proven, one thing I know is that the cancer survivors I've met who get involved with sustainable nourishment from seed to table improve their quality of life. Why? It's all about control. Cancer rips control from one's grasp, as life decisions and perhaps life's course are turned over to strangers. Even after the initial chaos passes, one doesn't hit the ground running but rather struggles on unsteady feet. In this context, engaging in sustainable nourishment is like taking part in a daily improvisational play that builds confidence. You can awake each morning and answer a question that too few of us ask: "What can I do for myself today that will be good for me?" In the course of just a few hours, a nourishing meal goes from inspiration to reality as one shops, preps, and cooks, not just for themselves, but for those they love as well. This experience, though it sounds hippie-ish to say so, can truly be transformative.

The key is finding the time and energy. My suggestion: If you can, find people to help. Friends and family are a good place to start, but remember that people who pitch in when times are tough don't necessarily want to make a culinary shift. Yes, they'll eat what you make them, and the delicious food may pique their interest, but I still suggest finding a cooking partner or two in the community. Such cooking buddies are probably as motivated as you are to shop, cook, and even clean. If possible, find someone who is an experienced cook. Their knowledge will accelerate your own development in the kitchen.

As for finding time, again I have a few suggestions. Many people like having a massive cook-a-thon on weekends, especially on Sunday. Once they get the routine down, my clients say they can cook, freeze, and refrigerate enough food to give them nutritious meals for the rest of the week. One day on, six days off? Sounds good to me. My friend says it also gave his two children a sense of responsibility for their own nutrition and health; they chose what they wanted to eat (healthy food, of course), cooked it, and put it in individually sized containers to be eaten later in the week.

I'm also a realist. Not everyone wants to completely change how they eat. I'm reminded of one of my grandmother's favorite sayings: "Everything in moderation . . . including moderation." Taking part in sustainable nourishment doesn't have to be an all-consuming affair. I'd rather someone enjoy getting together once a month with a cooking partner and making a great meal from scratch than to have them feel as if—oy!—they're on a burdensome diet. Remember, this is supposed to be fun! Make it a challenge—something that you want to do for yourself. Think of it as a personal contract where you get to choose the terms for nourishing yourself. Sometimes that contract need say nothing more than "Today, I'm going to eat to fit my needs."

For my client Andrea, that means thinking about her day's activities and eating accordingly. If she's going for a hike, she'll add a little extra protein for energy. If not, she'll eat light. Andrea also thinks of what's in her gas tank with regards to eating fresh and organic foods. She takes a pragmatic approach. "I only have a certain amount of energy. That's true even for healthy people," she says. "I can choose to use that energy fighting off toxins [in foods], or I can choose to use my energy to go kayaking. It always seems to be a much better proposition to eat well and be out in the world."

Learning about organic foods is also part of sustainable nourishment, but it's much more fun to learn about the subject from the ground up. The best classroom I know is the farmers' market. It's such a blast to go there. The farmers are delightful—talk about your salt-of-the-earth types! They love talking about what they grow and how they grow it. They're always chatting about what's at the height of season, and what's ready to be picked and brought to market in the next few weeks. If you really want to make their day, give them a recipe of something you've done with their food. Even if there's nothing in particular you want to buy, the food is so vibrant and the smells are so delightful that a trip down to the market is a guaranteed pick-me-up.

I'd also encourage subscribing to a few food magazines to stimulate your nourishment consciousness. Some contain many recipes, while others specialize in culinary reportage. And as your knowledge about and experience with sustainable nourishment expands, don't be surprised if you feel a desire to nourish others. You might even want to host a dinner party. This may come as quite a shock to those who've never initiated such social interactions, but I say go for it. Think of it as a tremendous opportunity to share a gift of life. That's what I call sustenance.

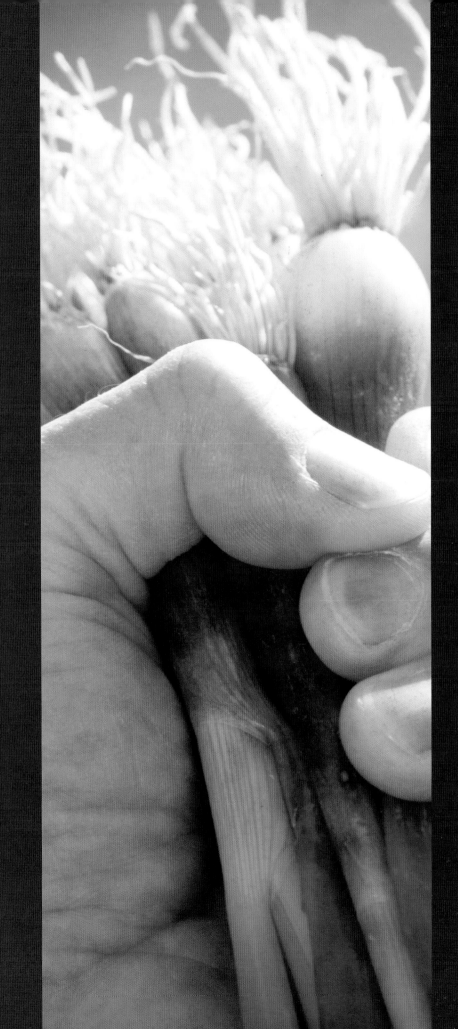

The benefit from cooking with whole foods—that is, foods that still retain their nutritional value versus their nutritionally stripped-down commercial cousins (think whole potatoes versus bagged potato chips with their preservatives, or a whole apple versus pasteurized apple juice)—is that you control what ingredients go into a dish. In effect, you become your own food processor. When you purchase highly processed foods, you don't have that control.

THE RECIPES IN THIS BOOK ARE ALL ABOUT DISCOVERING THE HEALTHIEST, TASTIEST FOODS OUT THERE THAT KEEP YOU WELL WHILE BATTLING CANCER. To that end, the nutritional analysis included with each recipe will give you an in-depth look at the macro-nutrient value of each dish; by *macro* we mean fat, carbohydrates, and protein . . . your body's major sources of fuel. By contrast, the Nutrition at a Glance table beginning on the opposite page covers the micro-nutrients found in each food used in this book—including the vitamins, minerals, and phytochemicals (*phyto* is Greek for 'plant-derived') that support the immune system and fight cancer.

I think of these analyses and tables as tools that can be used many ways, depending on an individual's needs. Often patients lose weight during treatments; for these people, knowing the amount of calories they're consuming in each dish is important. Sometimes the simplest way to gain weight is to double up on a portion. (And, speaking of portion size, a good rule of thumb is that a portion of poultry, fish, or meat is roughly the size of your fist, while a portion of vegetable or fruit is about the size of your full open hand.) If you're really not hungry, look for recipes that are higher in fat, as fat has a higher caloric count per gram than carbohydrates or proteins. Protein counts are also important to be aware of; because chemotherapy drains the body of protein, you'll need more than your usual share to boost immunity and ward off infection.

Regarding carbohydrates and fats, here are a few thoughts to consider. The more complex a carbohydrate, the more slowly it breaks down and delivers its sugars to your blood, which leads to better blood sugar control. Complex carbohydrates are typically found in the vegetables, legumes, and whole grains included in my recipes. Simple carbohydrates—think straight table sugar and most white grain, flour, and rice products—should be avoided because they dump a lot of sugar into your system very quickly.

Fats are also complex, in that all fats are not created equal. Some sit in the body like lumps of clay, while others are burned quickly and efficiently. The fats used in this book are the healthiest I could find, specifically olive oil and coconut milk/oil and the fat found in certain nuts and seeds, such as flaxseed. Used properly and judiciously, these fats offer wonderful benefits to cells and the immune system.

What you won't find in the nutritional analyses is the amount of sugars in each dish. That's because there is no added sugar in these recipes. There's no need, as the ingredients themselves release natural sugars that are well-balanced with healthy fats, protein, and fiber to keep insulin levels in check. The only exceptions to this are the recipes where I call for a smidge of Grade B organic maple syrup, but I've made sure to include more fiber in those recipes so the syrup's sugars are absorbed slowly and properly into the system.

I've always felt that, when it comes to nutrition, knowledge is power. Here's to a little enlightenment!

Nutrition at a Glance

We've scoured websites, scientific journals, the USDA's research, and reference books to come up with the following list of nutritional nuggets. Use them to impress your friends, or just to feel better about what you're putting in your body.

Recipe Element	Recipes to Live For	Nutritional Profile
Almonds	Almond Chocolate Chip Cookies (p. 103) Flourless Almond Torte (p. 108) Spiced Roasted Almonds (p. 99)	Essential food for maintaining or gaining weight. High fat, carbohydrate, and protein content. Rich in vitamin E and calcium. Easy to digest when finely ground.
Apples	Kabocha and Butternut Squash Soup (p. 22) Chicken Patties with Apple and Arugula (p. 51)	Apples are a major dietary source of an antioxidant phytochemical called quercetin. Quercetin benefits may include cancer protection, allergy symptom relief, and anticlotting effects.
Arugula	Basil and Arugula Pesto (p. 115) Mixed Greens with Roasted Beets and Avocado (p. 42)	Stimulates appetite and digestion. May reduce stomach and colon cramps.
Asparagus	Asparagus Soup with Pistachio Cream (p. 15)	Asparagus contains several important amino acids. Aspargine helps kidneys break down and excrete uric acid. Aspartic acid neutralizes excess ammonia, which causes fatigue. Asparagus' high water content and roughage encourages bowel activity.
Avocado	Avocado Cream (p. 115)	Good iron and copper content that protects against anemia by promoting red blood cell generation. Rich in glutathione, a powerful antioxidant that blocks absorption of certain unhealthy fats. Easily digested.
Bananas	Smoothies (pp. 97 and 98)	Provides substantial amounts of potassium, a mineral that is lost during bouts of physical activity, yet is vital for controlling the body's fluid balance. An excellent source of vitamin B_6 and a soluble fiber called pectin, which helps to lower LDL "bad" cholesterol levels. Soothes the stomach.
Basil, Cilantro, Mint	Everywhere!	Green herbs contain varying amounts of carotenoids, insoluble fibers, and an array of vitamins and minerals. Notably, fresh mint, chives, and parsley offer some folate, and $1/4$ cup of chopped parsley furnishes more than 20% of the daily requirements of vitamin C.
Beans	Black Bean Chili (p. 28) Black Bean Medley (p. 85) Tuscan Bean Soup with Kale (p. 27)	Studies suggest bean consumption may reduce cholesterol and regulate blood sugar. Also linked to lower rates of prostate and breast cancer.
Beets	Mixed Greens with Roasted Beets and Avocado (p. 42)	Beets help to dissolve and eliminate acid crystals from the kidneys. Also aids in reducing blood and organ toxins, especially in the liver and gallbladder.
Berries	Fruit Crisp (p. 105) Fruit Parfait with Almond-Peach-Ginger Cream (p. 112)	Contain ellagic acid, a potent antioxidant that is not heat sensitive. Blueberries contain more disease-fighting antioxidants than practically any other fruit or vegetable.
Bok Choy	Baby Bok Choy with Sesame and Ginger (p. 31) Stir-Fry Sauce with Vegetables (p. 45)	Bok choy contains high amounts of beta-carotene, vitamin B_6, vitamin C, folate, calcium, and iron.
Broccoli	Broccoli Sautéed with Garlic (p. 34) Szechwan Broccoli (p. 35) Emerald City Soup (p. 17)	Rich in cancer-fighting vitamins and phytochemicals. Excellent source of B vitamins, folate, riboflavin, potassium, iron, and vitamin C. Cooking increases vitamin absorption. The phytochemical sulforaphane inhibits the damaging effects of cancer-causing substances. Another chemical, dithiolthione, is believed to activate cancer-fighting enzymes in the body. May help metabolize excess estrogen, perhaps helping to prevent hormone-related tumors such as breast cancer. Raw broccoli contains almost as much calcium as whole milk.
Cabbage	Jicama and Red Cabbage Salad (p. 38)	Raw cabbage promotes waste elimination. Has alkaline properties, which some researchers believe may have cancer-preventive effects. Promotes nutrient absorption and growth of healthful intestinal flora. One study showed that eating cabbage more than once a week cut male colon cancer risk by nearly two-thirds.

continues

Recipe Element	Recipes to Live For	Nutritional Profile
Carrots	Carrot-Ginger Soup with Cashew Cream (p. 16) Magic Mineral Broth (p. 13)	Outstanding source of the antioxidant beta-carotene. Beta-carotene consumption is linked to reducing the risk of cancer, heart attacks, and cataracts. Other vitamins, minerals, and enzymes in carrots support liver, digestive, and kidney function.
Cashews	Anytime Crunch (p. 83) Cashew Tart Crusts (p. 106)	Good source of iron, magnesium, vitamin E, and zinc. Zinc loss, a common side effect of cancer treatments, may cause impaired taste.
Celery	Magic Mineral Broth (p. 13)	High in certain anticancer compounds that have been shown to detoxify carcinogens, including cigarette smoke. Tests show that celery may act as a mild diuretic.
Chicken	Chicken Patties with Apple and Arugula (p. 51) Chicken Potpie (p. 68) Chicken Soup with Bowtie Pasta (p. 11) Chicken Stew from My Nana (p. 24) All-Purpose Chicken Stock (p. 9) Chicken . . . Roasted All the Way to Yum! (p. 52) Lemony Chicken with Capers and Kalamata Olives (p. 54)	One 5-ounce serving of organic chicken provides 35 grams of easily digested protein. Excellent protein source for people with poor appetites. Contains the amino acid tyrosine, which the brain uses to produce substances (dopamine and norepinephrine) that enhance mental alertness.
Chickpeas	Chickpea Soup with Caramelized Fennel and Orange Zest (p. 12)	High in protein. Helps reduce blood cholesterol, control insulin and blood sugar, lower blood pressure, and regulate colon function.
Chili Peppers	Black Bean Chili (p. 26) Black Bean Medley (p. 85) Salsa Cruda (p. 121)	Revs up the blood clot–dissolving system, opens sinus and air passages, and acts as a decongestant. The benefits are credited to capsaicin, the compound that makes the pepper taste hot. Antioxidant or interferes with cancer development.
Cinnamon	Many!	A strong stimulator of insulin activity, thus potentially helpful for those with adult-onset diabetes. Also seems to help prevent blood clots.
Citrus Fruit	Fruit Crisp (p. 105) Fruit Parfait with Almond-Peach-Ginger Cream (p. 112)	The antioxidant actions of citrus flavonoids may counter unhealthy free radicals that contribute to diseases.
Coconut Milk/ Coconut Oil	Sweet Potato–Coconut Soup (p. 18) Poached Coconut Ginger Salmon (p. 59) Creamy Banana-Coconut Shake (p. 98)	Coconut milk is similar in chemical properties to mother's milk. Contains a form of lauric acid that fights viruses and bacteria. Supports the immune system.
Corn/Cornmeal	Stacked Polenta Pie (p. 80) Cornmeal Pizza (p. 92)	Corn is high in anticancer compounds called protease inhibitors. Fresh corn contains more enzymes and vitamins than dried varieties. High in fiber. Helps build bone and muscle. Excellent food for the brain and nervous system. May fight heart disease.
Couscous	Seasonal Couscous (p. 76)	Whole wheat couscous is rich in flavonoids, lignans, and saponins. Provides protein and B vitamins.
Eggs	Frittata with Herby Potatoes (p. 93) Tortilla Stack with Salsa Cruda (p. 62)	High in protein. Important source of vitamin B_{12}, riboflavin, and selenium. Egg white is almost pure protein, packed with amino acids. Egg yolks contain vitamins A and D. Eggs also contain lutein and zeaxanthin, which may have antioxidant properties.
Flax seeds	Smoothies (pp. 97 and 98)	Provides alpha-linolenic acids (ALA), which the body converts to omega-3 like fatty acids found mainly in fish. Such fatty acids may reduce the inflammatory process suspected in several cancers. Also high in fiber and antioxidants.
Fruit, Dried Prunes, Apricots, Cherries, Raisins and so on	Fruit Compote (p. 116)	Dried prunes are a high-fiber food. Over half of this fiber is easily assimilated by the body. Fiber lowers cholesterol. Nutrients in prunes include beta-carotene, iron, calcium, potassium, and selenium. Well-known to have a gentle laxative effect.

Recipe Element	Recipes to Live For	Nutritional Profile
Ginger	Ginger Ale/Ginger Tea (p. 94) Gingerbread (p. 111)	World's oldest and most popular medicinal spice. Promotes circulation and energy. Aids in digestion and assimilation of food. May ease cold or flu symptoms. Also relieves some inflammatory pain and swelling.
Jicama	Jicama and Red Cabbage Salad with Mint and Cilantro (p. 38)	High in fiber, potassium, iron, calcium, and A, B-complex, and C vitamins. Low fat.
Kale	Dark Leafy Greens with Caramelized Onions, Raisins, and Pine Nuts (p. 36) Delicata Squash with Dino Kale and Cranberries (p. 41) Emerald City Soup (p. 17)	A cruciferous vegetable rich in calcium and cancer-fighting compounds, including antioxidants. Sulforaphane, also in broccoli, is a well-studied phytochemical that may inhibit cancer-causing substances. Other kale phytochemicals may protect against breast cancer by reducing the impact of estrogen. Beneficial to the function of the digestive and nervous systems.
Lentils	Lemony Lentil Soup with Pistachio Mint Pesto (p. 25)	Easily digested. A rich supply of minerals for organs, glands, and tissues.
Lettuce and Mixed Salad Greens	My Favorite Salad (p. 44) Mixed Greens with Roasted Beets and Avocado (p. 42)	Large organic water content. Contains nearly all the necessary vitamins to sustain health. High in silicon, which helps renew joints, bones, arteries, and connective tissue. Greener and darker leaves are more nutritious.
Miso	Miso-Ginger Soup with Udon Noodles (p. 14)	Miso should be used in moderation because of high sodium content (900 milligrams per tablespoon). Made from a combination of soybeans and grains such as rice or barley.
Oats	Best Oatmeal Ever (p. 84) Anytime Crunch (p. 83)	Higher proportion of fat and protein than other grains. Contains antioxidants, iron, and zinc. Zinc consumption is often important for people whose taste buds have been impaired by cancer treatments. High fiber content has mild laxative effect. Rich silicon properties help renew bones and connective tissue.
Olive Oil, Dulse Flakes	Lemon Caper Vinaigrette (p. 119) Sea-ser Dressing (p. 122)	An important source of the phytochemicals hydroxytyrosol and oleuropein. These substances are being studied because of their antioxidant properties and potential to protect against breast cancer, clogged arteries, and high blood pressure.
Onions/Leeks	Caramelized Sweet Red Onion Soup with Parmesan Crostini (p. 10) Yukon Gold Potato Leek Soup (p. 23) Magic Mineral Broth (p. 13)	Onions: A rich source of the phytochemical diallyl sulfide. May increase protective enzymes that help to inactivate and eliminate cancer-causing agents. Leeks: A good source of fiber and iron. Low in calories.
Oranges	Chickpea Soup with Caramelized Fennel and Orange Zest (p. 12) Pecans Spiced with Orange Zest and Ginger (p. 95)	A complete package of cancer inhibitors, including antioxidants such as vitamin C. Specifically tied to lower rates of pancreatic cancer. Because of their high vitamin C content, oranges may also help ward off breast and stomach cancer, asthma attacks, atherosclerosis, and gum disease.
Papaya	Fruit and Fresh Herb Salsa (p. 122)	An excellent source of vitamin C. Also contains fiber, folate, vitamin E, potassium, and beta-carotene.
Parsley	Grandma Nora's Salsa Verde (p. 117) Magic Mineral Broth (p. 13)	Green herbs, most notably parsley, fresh mint, and chives, contain an array of vitamins and minerals. A quarter cup of chopped parsley furnishes more than 20% of the daily requirement of vitamin C. Chlorophyll freshens breath.
Pecans	Pecans Spiced with Orange Zest and Ginger (p. 95) Anytime Crunch (p. 83)	High in thiamine, zinc, and fiber. Boosts the immune system. Zinc rebuilds damaged taste buds.
Potatoes	Mashed Yukon Gold Potatoes with Rutabaga (p. 73) Magic Mineral Broth (p. 13)	Extremely nutritional vegetable. Contains complex carbohydrates along with proteins, vitamins, and minerals such as vitamin B_6, vitamin C, potassium, and iron. Potato skins are a rich source of fiber.

continues

Recipe Element	Recipes to Live For	Nutritional Profile
Quinoa	Couscous Quinoa with Mint and Tomatoes (p. 67)	High-energy protein. Eases digestion. Gluten free, which makes it an important food for those with wheat allergies. More calcium than milk. Higher in fat content than most grains. Rich in minerals.
Rice	Coconut-Ginger Rice with Cilantro (p. 100) Asian Japonica Rice Salad with Edamame (p. 90)	Brown Rice: Milling process removes only hulls, leaving rice high in B-complex and E vitamins, magnesium, and potassium. White Rice: Milled to remove entire husk. Significantly less dietary fiber than brown rice. Helps treat diarrhea.
Salmon	Miso Salmon with Lime-Ginger Glaze (p. 60) Poached Coconut Ginger Salmon (p. 59)	Excellent source of protein. High in omega-3 fatty acids. These acids may reduce inflammation suspected of playing a role in the development of certain cancers and heart disease. Salmon also contains a form of iron that is easily absorbed. A good source of B vitamins, thiamine, niacin, and vitamin D.
Soy/Tofu	Sweet "Ricotta" (p. 123) Veggie "Ricotta" Lasagna (p. 77) Herbed "Ricotta" (p. 118)	Excellent cancer fighter. Contains omega-3 fatty acids, which may reduce inflammation implicated in the development of certain cancers. Phytochemicals called isoflavones may act as antioxidants and have beneficial effects on cholesterol, cardiovascular health, and the brain. Helps regulate insulin and blood sugar levels. Good protein builder. Contains eight essential amino acids.
Spinach	Spinach Orzo with Pine Nuts and Feta (p. 78)	High in vitamins and minerals, including B_6, folate, magnesium, and riboflavin. Rich in carotenoids, including beta-carotene, lutein, and zeaxanthin. Cooking spinach with a small amount of olive oil enhances absorption of fat-soluble carotenoids. Also rich in chlorophyll.
Squash	Kabocha and Butternut Squash Soup (p. 22) Delicata Squash with Dino Kale and Cranberries (p. 41) Baby Dumpling Squash Stuffed with Rice Medley (p. 33)	Packed with nutrition and one of the easiest vegetables to digest. May help reduce inflammation. Strengthens the immune system. High in beta-carotene, vitamins C and E, folate, iron, and magnesium.
String Beans	String Beans with Caramelized Shallots, Rosemary, and Garlic (p. 46) Bombay Beans (p. 47)	Abundant in potassium, which benefits the heart, pancreas, and salivary glands. Yellow or wax beans are considered inferior to the green bean in nutritional value.
Sweet Potatoes	Mashed Ginger Sweet Potatoes with Fresh Nutmeg (p. 72) Magic Mineral Broth (p. 13) Sweet Potato–Coconut Soup (p. 18)	Actually an edible root unrelated to the potato. Excellent nutritional profile. High in fiber, vitamins B_6 and C, iron, and potassium.
Swiss Chard	Swiss Chard Pasta (p. 75) Swiss Chard "Ricotta" Galettes (p. 87) Swiss Chard Braised with Sweet Tomatoes and Corn (p. 40) Garlicky Leafy Greens (p. 37)	A rich source of beta-carotene and potassium. Supplies fiber, vitamins C and E, and magnesium. Extremely rich in vitamin K, which is essential for bone formation.
Tomatoes	Taxicab Yellow Tomato Soup with Fresh Basil Pesto (p. 21) Puttanesca Sauce (p. 120) Salsa Cruda (p. 121)	A major source of the antioxidant lycopene. Tomato consumption has been linked to lower rates of bladder, breast, prostate, and colorectal cancer. Cooking with an oil may increase the absorption of lycopene.
Turkey	Turkey Patties (p. 61)	Rich in amino acids that build proteins. Source of L-trytophan, which can have a relaxing effect. Helps production of serotonin, a mood regulator. Dark meat contains almost three times as much iron as white meat.
Whey or Soy Protein Powder	Smoothies (pp. 97 and 98)	Protein powder contains a complete amino acid profile. One scoop of powder provides 16 grams of protein. Good for people having a hard time getting enough protein in their diet due to loss of appetite.

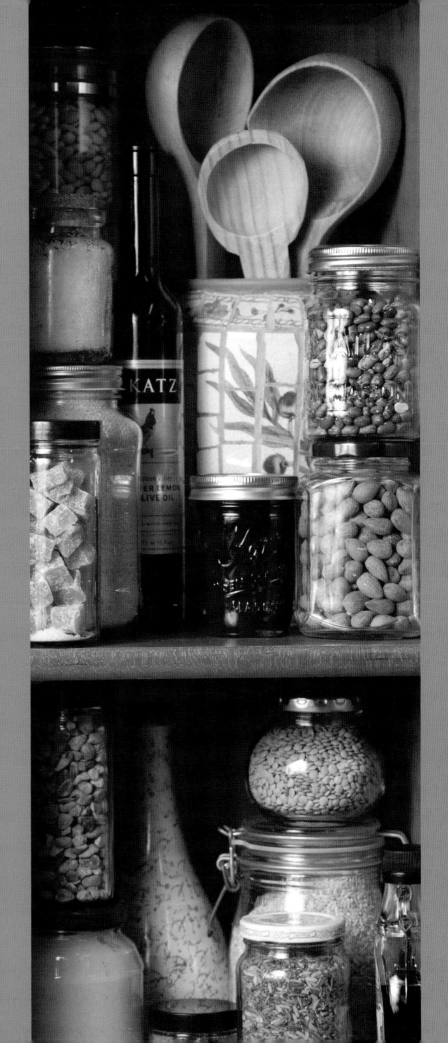

Get out those garbage bags. Put the dog in another room. Tell the kids to go in the den and watch a rerun of Saved by the Bell. It's time to get down to some serious business: We're going to clean out the pantry!

TO BE AN EFFECTIVE, EFFICIENT COOK, YOU HAVE TO HAVE THE RIGHT TOOLS FOR THE JOB. THE TOOLBOX? THAT'S YOUR PANTRY. This chapter lists everything you'll need, from food staples to utensils, to make your kitchen a lean, mean, culinary machine. Each item is thoroughly explained, and a list organizes the items according to where you can expect to find them in the market. A final section emphasizes the impor-tance of shopping for organics.

Pantry Staples

AGAR AGAR: Also called *kanten*, this tasteless dried seaweed can replace gelatin in recipes. It's sold packaged in powdered form at natural food stores and Asian markets.

BROWN RICE VINEGAR: Its light, clean taste adds a mild acidity to foods. Used in salad dressings and marinades.

COCONUT OIL: A healthier saturated fat. It's made up of medium-chain triglycerides (MCTs) that are converted into energy and are not stored in the body as fat. Coconut oil is nutritious, easily digestible, and withstands high levels of heat without becoming an unhealthy trans-fatty acid. It is used for baking and stove-top cooking. For those avoiding dairy, coconut oil is a great alternative to butter.

CORNMEAL: Dried corn that has been ground into a coarse flour. Used for breads. Also called polenta.

DULSE FLAKES: A red, salty seaweed that is excellent for sprinkling on many greens, including salads. Like most sea vegetables, dulse is high in iron, iodine, and manganese. Available in most natural food stores. Look for Sea Seasonings Organic Dulse Granules produced by Maine Coast Sea Vegetables.

EDAMAME: Fresh young soybeans in green pods. Available fresh from June through October. A good snack straight from the pod. Cascadian Farms has frozen packages throughout the year.

FLOUR: Any grain can be ground into flour. We suggest organic unbleached all-purpose white flour, which is less refined than commercial white flour, for general use. Flour should be bought fresh and stored in airtight containers in either a refrigerator or a cool, dark space.

HERBS AND SPICES: Herbs are the fragrant leaves of annual or perennial plants that grow in temperate zones. Common herbs include basil, bay leaf, chervil, marjoram, mint, oregano, parsley, rosemary, sage, savory, tarragon, and thyme. Spices are pungent or aromatic seasonings obtained from the bark, buds, fruit, roots, seeds, or stems of plants and trees. Herbs and spices should be kept in airtight containers away from light and heat. Use within a year for maximum flavor. Try to buy organic herbs.

KAFFIR LIME LEAVES: From the kaffir or wild lime tree, the leaves have a very pungent, limelike scent. Available fresh, frozen, or dried. When purchased fresh they keep in the freezer for months. Most commonly used in Thai cooking like a bay leaf. Can be found at Asian specialty markets.

KOMBU: Long, dark brown to black seaweed that is dried and folded into sheets. Keeps indefinitely when stored in a cool, dry place. Kombu contains a full range of trace minerals often deficient in people with compromised immune systems. High in potassium, iodine, calcium, and vitamins A and C.

KUDZU OR KUZU: A root starch pulverized into a powder. Used to thicken soups and sauces or as a substitute for cornstarch or arrowroot. The powder must be dissolved in cold water before being added to food. Kudzu has calming properties that aid digestion.

MAPLE SYRUP (Grade B Organic): Darker and richer than its Grade A cousin, it's also not quite as sweet. A small amount of Grade B maple syrup imparts a cozy, full flavor to food. Excellent for baking and cooking. Buy only organic maple syrup, as non-organic brands may use formaldehyde and other chemicals.

MIRIN: A Japanese sweet rice wine that adds sweetness and gentle flavor to sauces and dressings. I partner it with tamari, ginger, garlic, and sesame oils. Mirin is available without additives in most natural food stores.

MISO: Also called bean paste, this Japanese culinary mainstay has the consistency of peanut butter. Miso is used in sauces, soups, marinades, and salad dressings. The lighter the color of miso, the mellower it is: white (made with rice) is smooth, red is richer, and dark brown is full-bodied and salty. Miso is extremely nutritious. Store tightly covered in the fridge. Use within three months.

NORI: Paper-thin sheets of dried seaweed. It has a sweet and salty taste that partners well with roasted nuts. Rich in protein, calcium, iron, and trace minerals. Commonly used to wrap sushi.

OLIVE OIL (extra virgin): An ancient oil still pressed from tree-ripened olives. Considered a healthy source of fat. There are many types of olive oil, but I prefer using cold-pressed, which means the oil was made without heat or chemical treatments. Store large quantities of olive oil in a cool, dark place; keep your everyday supply in a dark container. Use within six months. Buy organic, if possible.

RAPADURA: Unrefined whole organic sugar that has a unique caramel taste and natural coloring. Offers nutritional value far superior to that of refined sugar. Captures the sweet essence of evaporated sugar cane. Use in the same proportions as refined sugar . . . meaning use it sparingly!

RICE (basmati): A long-grain rice imported from India. *Basmati* translates as "queen of fragrance." Basmati is chewy and light in texture and has a nutty aroma. Available in white or brown.

RICE (jasmine): An aromatic rice originally from Thailand. It has a nutty flavor similar to basmati rice.

SAFFLOWER OIL: This flavorless, colorless oil extracted from safflower seeds is healthier than vegetable oils such as corn oil. I strongly recommend using Spectrum brand's 100 percent expeller-pressed unrefined organic safflower oil. It is made without hexane or other harmful chemicals. Keep refrigerated after opening.

SEA SALT: Salt garnered from the natural evaporation of seawater. It's far healthier than common iodized table salt and contains more than eighty valuable trace minerals. Available in fine grains or larger crystals.

SESAME OIL: Oil pressed from the sesame seed. The lighter version is very mild and good for cooking, as it resists breaking down under heat. The darker version, called toasted sesame oil, has a strong, nutty flavor. It is heat-sensitive, so use it sparingly to flavor Asian-style dishes that are off the flame. If these oils are packaged in clear glass bottles, try to purchase bottles from the back of the shelf that have not been exposed to much light (this is true for the purchase of all oils).

SPELT FLOUR: Has a mellow, nutty flavor and a slightly higher protein content than wheat. For people sensitive to wheat, the gluten contained in spelt may be easier to digest.

STOCK: Keep a few 1-quart boxes handy in your pantry for when you don't have time to make home-made stock. Purchase organic vegetable or chicken stock made by Pacific or Imagine.

SUNFLOWER OIL: A flavorless all-purpose oil with a fatty acid profile similar to that of extra virgin olive oil. Perfect for baking and cooking over medium heat. This oil can be substituted in all baking recipes for any vegetable oil. I recommend High-O Sunflower Oil Blend by Omega Nutrition.

TAMARI: A dark sauce made from soybeans. The taste is similar to that of soy sauce, but tamari is made without wheat.

TOFU: Made from fermented soybean milk, tofu comes in soft, medium, and firm varieties. Sold packaged in water. Keep refrigerated; it's extremely perishable. Tofu is rich in protein and low in fat.

UDON NOODLES: These Japanese noodles of varying thicknesses are made from wheat flour. Sold fresh and dried.

WORCESTERSHIRE SAUCE: This thin, dark, and piquant sauce is used to season everything from vegetable juices (it goes extremely well with tomato) to sauces, soups, and salad dressings. It's now available in organic and vegetarian varieties.

Food Storage

Foods that are exposed or stored at room temperature can develop bacteria and mold. Store hot foods in sealable plastic containers as soon as they cool down. Keep on hand airtight containers in several sizes with indented lids: These seal well, exclude air, and facilitate stacking. Use masking tape and a permanent marker to label containers with the date and contents (this makes it easy to identify and toss outdated food before it becomes a science experiment). Glass storage jars are not necessarily airtight.

Use vegetables as soon as possible after purchase. Storing them too long robs them of freshness and sweetness. Don't wash vegetables until you are ready to use them; they will last longer if not washed in advance. Place vegetables in the crisper drawer in the refrigerator. Keep lettuces in a resealable plastic bag with a paper towel inside to absorb moisture. Poke a couple of holes in the bag.

When storing food in aluminum foil, I recommend cutting a piece of parchment paper slightly smaller than the piece of foil. Place the parchment on the foil, then place the food on the parchment and wrap. This keeps the food from coming in contact with the foil, avoiding the possibility of the foil leaching into and reacting to the acids in the food.

Good Things to Have in Your Freezer!

Magic Mineral Broth (page 13)
Stocks (pages 9 and 53)
Roasted tomatoes (page 120)
Nuts
Various roasted nuts (page 151)
Pestos (pages 25 and 115)
Grandma Nora's Salsa Verde (page 117)
Frozen fruit
Fruit Compote (page 116)

Kitchen Equipment Checklist

BAKING DISHES: Choose convenient sizes and styles. Common types include an 8- or 9-inch square glass or ceramic baking dish, a 9-inch tart pan with removable bottom, an 8- to 10-inch springform pan, and a 9- or 10-inch glass or ceramic pie plate.

BAKING SHEETS: There are two types of baking sheets—a flat cookie sheet and a sheet pan or jellyroll pan that has raised sides. Always use the rimmed pan for roasting so juices or oils don't spill and force you to clean the oven. Common sizes are 14 by 17 inches or 12 by 17 inches. Before you buy, measure the interior of your oven!

BLENDER: Great for making silky smooth soups, sauces, nut creams, and smooooothies. A word of caution when blending hot liquids: To avoid splatter burns and liquid dripping down the wall, don't fill the blender past the two-thirds mark. Also, put a towel over the lid before starting the blender. A blender's tall, narrow, leak-proof container is preferable to a food processor when blending liquids. Blending also adds air, resulting in a lighter finished product. (See also Vita-Mix.)

BOWLS: Use lightweight nesting stainless-steel bowls. They're easy to maintain, durable, and inexpensive, so you can keep every size on hand.

CHEESECLOTH: Use unbleached cheesecloth to strain soups and stocks or to tie herbs into a small bundle to use in soups and stews.

CHINOIS AND PESTLE: A cone-shaped mesh sieve used to remove sediment from stocks and make sauces velvety smooth. The pestle is tapered to fit into the bottom of the sieve to help push liquids through.

COLANDER: Should have wide grips for easy lifting or for resting the colander on a bowl or pot. Widely spaced holes are designed to drain larger items such as pasta and potatoes. Available in a variety of sizes and hole diameters. Line your colander with cheesecloth before straining broths and stocks.

CUTTING BOARD: You have two choices here—the resin in natural wood boards is bacteria resistant, as long as the wood has not been treated, but plastic and polyethylene boards are dishwasher safe. Regardless of which material you choose, buy two boards. Use one exclusively for vegetables, the other for meat and poultry. Wash well after use.

FINE-MESH SIEVES: Small sieves are ideal for sifting flour and other fine powders. Use larger sieves for draining or blanching vegetables.

FOOD PROCESSOR: Choose a processor with at least an 11-cup container. The metal blade (S shaped) does everything from chopping vegetables to making cookie dough. Alternate blades are available for specific tasks. A mini food processor has a smaller bowl and motor and is good for nuts, pesto, salad dressings, and other small grinding jobs.

KNIVES: We recommend buying three knives. The most important is a sharp 8-inch chef's knife that you will use for most cutting and chopping. Also purchase a 2- to 3-inch paring knife for delicate slicing or paring and a 10-inch serrated bread knife. To keep your knives sharp—a sharp knife is much safer than a dull knife—you will need an item called a steel to hone the blade. A few swipes on the steel will do it!

LADLES: Essential for serving soups and sauces. Get a 6- to 8-ounce ladle for soups and a 2- to 4-ounce ladle for sauces.

LEMON SQUEEZER: My favorite kitchen toy disguised as a tool. This bright yellow handheld gadget takes a lemon or lime and, with one squeeze, extracts either all the juice or as little as you want.

MEASURING SPOONS AND CUPS: When scooping dry measurements, fill the measuring cup to overflowing and then level it off with a knife. Sets should include $1/8$-, $1/4$-, $1/3$-, and $1/2$-, and 1-cup measures. Stainless-steel items are best, but it's also good to have glass measuring cups in 1-cup to 1-quart sizes.

MEAT THERMOMETER: To get an accurate reading, place the tip of the thermometer close to the center of the meat. Digital thermometers are also available.

MICROPLANE GRATER: My second favorite kitchen toy! This indispensable tool is perfect for grating citrus zest, fresh whole nutmeg, or cheese. It comes in a variety of sizes and levels of coarseness.

MORTAR AND PESTLE: A small bowl with a slightly abrasive unglazed interior surface is used with a pestle to grind spices and seeds.

OVEN THERMOMETER: Don't trust that thirty-year-old temperature gauge on the oven. Why? Toasting at the wrong temperature can turn those almonds into dust. Check the accuracy of the oven's temperature before starting to bake.

PARCHMENT PAPER: Great for lining baking pans. Saves time and cleanup. For food storage, I recommend using a sheet of parchment between aluminum foil and the food to prevent the aluminum from leaching into and reacting with a food's acids.

POTS AND PANS: These generally come in six varieties: Sauce pots and pans, sauté pans, stockpots, roasting pans, grill pans, and frying pans. Heavy-bottomed pots and pans are essential. Stainless-steel 18/10 gauge is my pick. The base has an aluminum/magnetic steel core sealed between two layers of stainless steel. This is perfect for sound heat conduction and suitable for all stove tops.

Sauce pots and pans come in various sizes from 1 quart to $5^1/_2$ quarts. Sauté pans typically come in 8-, 10-, and 12-inch diameters. Pans with sloping sides are easier to use. Stockpots are usually 12 quarts and larger. When buying a roasting pan, consider a 10 by 15-inch pan, which is great for roasting a chicken. Grill pans, which come in one standard size, are most effective on a gas stove. They should be rubbed with oil before using. I suggest buying an 8-inch nonstick frying pan for cooking eggs. Make sure the pan is hot before add-ing the butter or oil. This will prevent the butter or oil from penetrating the nonstick surface. Use only nonmetal utensils with this pan. Avoid scouring and abrasive materials, and replace the pan if the coat-ing begins to crack or peel.

RUBBER SPATULA: Heat-resistant spatulas come in many sizes and colors.

SALAD SPINNER: For drying lettuce leaves or greens.

TIMER: Essential! Get one that rings loud enough to be heard in another room.

TONGS: Spring-action stainless-steel tongs act like extensions of your fingers and provide extra leverage and dexterity when handling hot foods. Use for turning roasted or grilled vegetables and meats. Available in 8- or 10-inch lengths, or even longer for deep pots and long reaches.

VEGETABLE PEELERS: Buy two sharp swivel peelers so a friend can help make those potato- and carrot-peeling jobs faster.

VITA-MIX: This multitasker blends and whips at warp speed and is a huge time-saver in my kitchen. An extremely powerful motor allows this machine to turn raw or cooked food into a silky purée. A kitchen dream come true!

WIRE WHISK: Used to incorporate air into food or smooth out lumps. There are a number of shapes, sizes, and weights. Choose stainless-steel whisks that fit comfortably in your hand.

WOODEN SPOONS: Unlike metal spoons, wood stays cool because it doesn't transfer heat. Have a number of sizes on hand for every task.

Seasonal Foods and Farmers' Markets

ONE OF THE PLEASURES OF COOKING IS ALWAYS HAVING FRESH INGREDIENTS AT HAND. As the seasons change, so do the foods the earth gives forth. It's enjoyable to look forward to a coming season, knowing that a favorite food (strawberries!) is about to make its annual debut at the farmers' market. Following is a general guide to what you may see at the farmers' market, depending upon the time of year. Remember that many staples are also available year-round at your supermarket, and some surprises are sure to show up at farmers' markets in different regions of the country. Still, the following overview will help you connect to the place where your food comes from: Mother Earth.

Anxiety-Free Shopping

The term *organic* typically describes food grown without chemicals, including fertilizers, insecticides, artificial coloring, artificial flavoring, and additives. For my money, organic food is the best: best for taste, best for color, best for health, and the best buy for your money. Growers and manufacturers can claim their foods are organic only if they meet the standards of the Federal Organic Foods Production Act and are certified by either state or federal officials. However, some small farmers who choose not to spend the money or time on such certification may still raise their foods, poultry, and meats without the use of any chemicals, hormones, or antibiotics. These farmers are often at farmers' markets and are usually glad to talk about the way they raise their products. Of course, without organic certification you're taking the farmer at their word.

Some fruits and vegetables should be avoided if they're not organically grown because the non-organic versions contain high levels of pesticides.

The Environmental Working Group recommends avoiding the following nonorganically raised produce:

Apples	Nectarines
Bell peppers	Peaches
Carrots	Pears
Celery	Potatoes
Cherries	Spinach
Grapes (imported)	Strawberries
Lettuce	

The following nonorganically raised fruits and vegetables have the least amount of pesticide residue:

Asparagus	Frozen sweet peas
Avocados	Kiwi
Bananas	Mangoes
Broccoli	Onions
Cabbage	Papaya
Cauliflower	Pineapples
Frozen sweet corn	

Season by Season

When shopping at the farmers' market, leave your shopping list at home. Instead, let your senses guide you. The chart on the next page, however, will give you an idea of some of the delights you'll find at the farmers' markets in various seasons. For more information on seasonal availability, check out the following web sites:

"What's Ripe Report" on www.epicurious.com/
    e02_ripe/ripe.html
www.eatwellguide.org
www.localharvest.com
www.ota.com
www.ams.usda.gov/farmersmarkets/map.html

Produce by Season

Spring

Apricots	Green garlic
Artichokes	Leeks
Arugula	Mangoes
Asparagus	Mixed baby greens
Avocados	Radishes
Beets	Rhubarb
Baby carrots	Shallots
Cauliflower	Spinach
Daikon	Strawberries
Dandelion greens	Sugar snap peas
Cherries	Swiss chard
Fava beans	Turnips
Fennel	Watercress

Summer

Blackberries	Peaches
Blueberries	Peppers
Corn	Plums
Cucumbers	String beans
Eggplant	Summer squashes
Figs	(zucchini, yellow
Melons	crookneck)
Nectarines	Tomatillos
Okra	Tomatoes

Fall

Apples	Hard-shelled
Arugula	squashes
Asian pears	(acorn squash,
Beans (cranberry	butternut, blue
and shell beans)	Hubbard, delicata,
Bell peppers	baby dumpling,
Broccoli	pumpkins)
Broccoli rabe	Pears
Brussels sprouts	Persimmons
Fennel	Pomegranates
Green tomatoes	Radicchio
	Sweet potatoes

Winter

Bok choy	Leeks
Cabbage	Parsnips
Celery root	Rainbow chard
Citrus fruits	Rutabagas
Collard greens	Swiss chard
Kale	

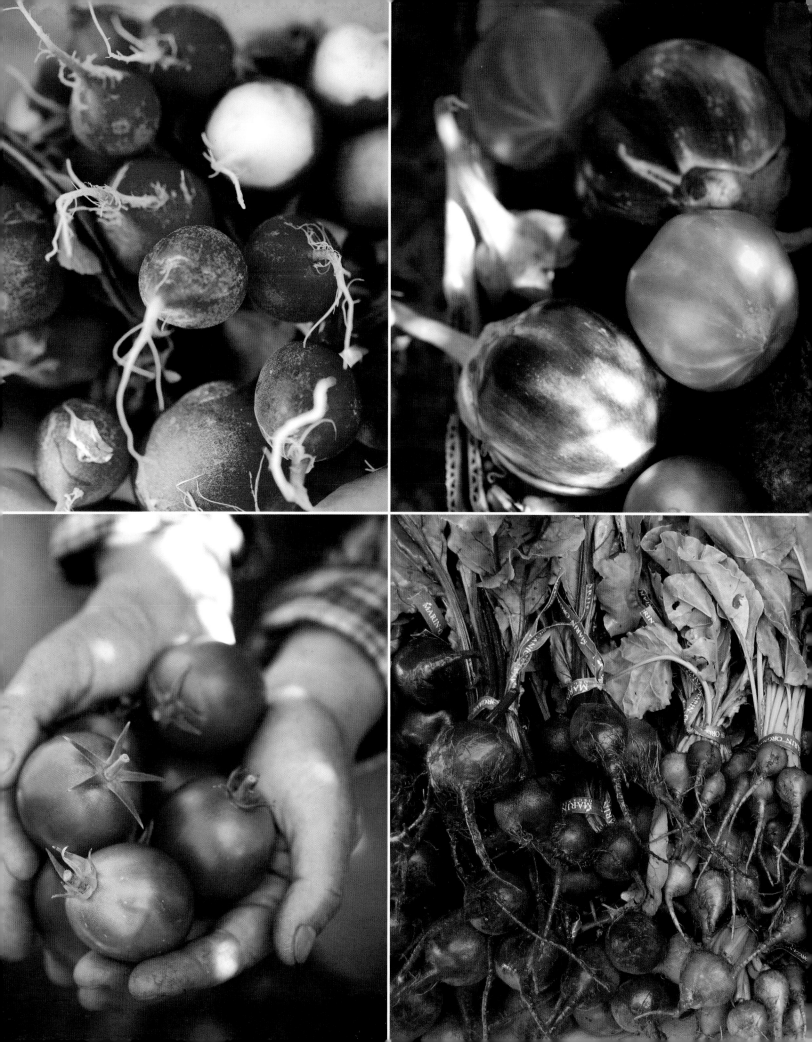

Pantry Rehabilitation

Remember to buy organic. Make copies of this chart to take with you while you shop.

Fresh
Edamame
Farmers' market greens
Garlic
Ginger
Jalapeños
Kaffir lime leaves
Lemongrass
Lemons
Limes
Onions/Shallots
Oranges
Seasonal herbs

Dairy
Blond miso
Eggs—Omega-3s
Tofu—*Wildwood*

Freezer
Fruit—*Cascadian Farms*

Bulk Section
All-purpose unbleached flour
Almonds, raw, blanched, sliced
Apricots, unsulfured
Cannellini beans, dried
Cashews, whole and pieces
Chickpeas (garbanzo beans)
Coconut, shredded

Rice/Grain/Pasta/Bread
Japonica rice—*Lundberg*
Brown basmati rice—*Lundberg*
Brown rice penne—*Lundberg*
Brown jasmine rice—*Lundberg*
Wild/Brown rice blend—*Lundberg*
Israeli couscous
Pasta and spelt pasta
Udon noodles
Rice noodles—*Annie Chun*
Sprouted breads—*Alvarado St.*
Cornmeal crusts—*Vicolo*

Couscous
Cranberries, dried
Currants
Lentils
Oats
Orzo
Pecans
Pine nuts
Pistachios
Polenta
Prunes
Quinoa
Raisins
Spelt flour
Sun-dried tomatoes, unsulfured
Walnuts

Packaged Dry Goods
Agar agar flakes
Chocolate chips—malt-
    sweetened—*Sunspire*
Dulse flakes
Kombu
Kudzu—*Eden*
Nori
Organic stocks—*Pacific* or *Imagine*
Rapadura—*Rapunzel*
Maple crystals

Jarred & Canned Foods
Sunflower Oil—*Omega Nutrition*
Extra virgin olive oil
Safflower oil—*Spectrum*
Toasted sesame oil–*Spectrum*
Brown rice vinegar—*Spectrum*
Sesame oil—*Spectrum*
Coconut butter and oil—*Omega
    Nutrition* or *Spectrum*
Tamari
Mirin—*Eden*
Tomatoes—*Muir Glen*
Garbanzo beans—*Eden*
Black beans—*Eden*

Cannellini—*Eden*
Coconut milk—*Thai Kitchen*
Capers
Olives—*Mediterranean*
Salmon (pink)—*Crown Prince*
Anchovies—*Crown Prince*
Almond butter
Peanut butter
Blackstrap molasses
Local honey
Grade B organic maple syrup

Spices & Herbs
Allspice, whole and ground
Almond extract
Baking powder
Baking soda
Basil
Bay leaves
Black peppercorns
Cayenne
Chili powder
Cinnamon, ground
Cinnamon sticks
Coriander
Cumin, seeds and ground
Curry powder
Fennel seeds
Ginger
Juniper berries
Nutmeg, whole
Oregano
Red pepper flakes
Rosemary
Saffron
Sage
Sea salt
Star anise
Thyme
Turmeric
Vanilla extract

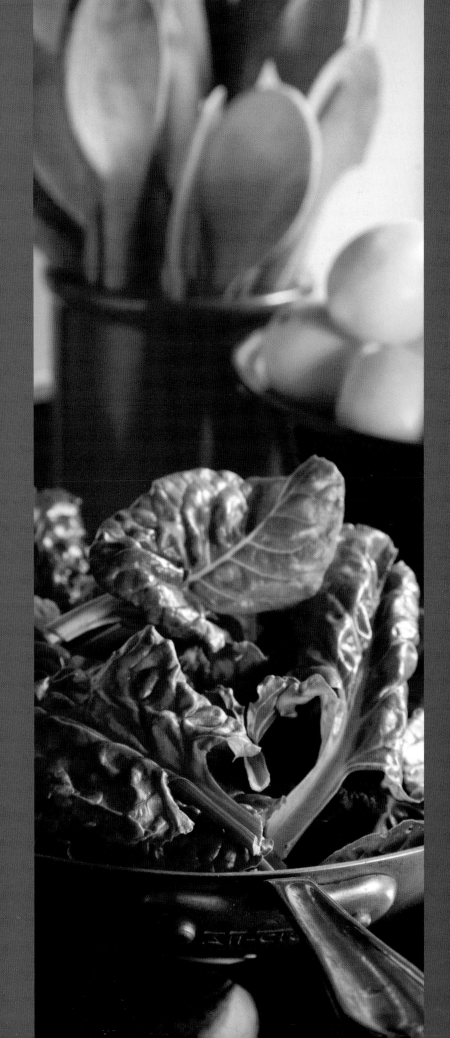

YOU CAN'T KNOW THE PLAYERS WITHOUT A
SCORECARD. HERE THE CULINARY TERMS USED
THROUGHOUT THIS BOOK ARE EXPLAINED.

Al dente
Italian for "to the tooth." This term describes how
pasta and many vegetables should be prepared.
"Al dente" foods are tender yet still slightly textured.

Beans
Beans are normally available in bulk or prepackaged.
One cup of dried beans yields two cups cooked. To
cook dried beans, sort out dirt and broken beans and
rinse the beans well in a strainer. Place in a bowl or
pot and cover with water (you may have to add more
water as the beans soak). Squeeze the juice of one
lemon into the soaking water (throw in the rind, too)
and refrigerate for at least 8 hours or overnight. Rinse
the soaked beans well before cooking. Soaking beans
breaks down the complex sugars (oligosaccharides)
that hinder digestion. I also always add kombu, a
sea vegetable, during the cooking process. Kombu
has a high mineral content that reduces the gas
produced by bean starch. Some canned beans, such
as Eden brand, include kombu. Rinse canned beans
well and wake up their flavor with a spritz of lemon
and a pinch of salt. Cooking times for beans vary
depending upon their variety and age, so taste often
during the cooking process. Place soaked and rinsed
beans in a pot, cover with 3 inches of water, and add
a 6-inch piece of kombu. Bring to a boil and decrease
the heat. Cook the beans at a low simmer (bubbles
will occasionally break the surface) for 45 minutes to
1 hour; begin tasting after 30 minutes. When the
beans are tender but still al dente, add 1 teaspoon
sea salt to the pot (adding salt too soon retards the
cooking process). The last 15 minutes are important,
as the beans start to cook faster; taste to ensure the
beans don't overcook. Drain, discard the water, and
rinse the beans with cold water. Proceed with the
recipe or, when completely cooled, store the beans
in an airtight container in your fridge or freezer.
Cooked beans can be frozen for up to 1 month. If you

are planning on storing and reheating beans, leave
them slightly undercooked.

Blanching
Partially cooking vegetables by plunging them
rapidly into boiling salted water. This heightens color,
especially for green vegetables. After blanching,
plunge the vegetables into a bowl of ice water to halt
the cooking process. This is also called a "cold water
bath" or "shocking."

Braising
Food is first browned in a fat (my choice is olive oil),
then cooked, tightly covered, in a small amount of
liquid at low heat for a long time. This slow cooking
develops flavor and tenderizes foods by gently
breaking down their fibers. Braise in an oven or on
top of a range.

Browning
The food's exterior browns while the interior
stays moist, giving food a rich flavor and lovely
color. This is accomplished by cooking quickly at
extremely high heat. Browning is usually done
on the stove.

Caramelizing Onions
This technique requires patience. During cooking,
onions slowly go through a number of visual stages,
from translucent to a deep golden brown, as they
release their yummy sugars. Keep in mind that
onions will cook down to less than one-third their
original volume as they are caramelized. Heat
2 tablespoons of olive oil in a large, heavy stainless-
steel sauté pan. Add the onions. Sprinkle with sea
salt; this helps the onions give up their juices. Sauté
briefly so all the onions have been exposed to the
heat and coated with oil. Decrease the heat to very
low and put down your spoon. Allow the onions
to cook slowly for 20 to 40 minutes (depending on
the number of onions). Do not stir! After about
20 minutes, the onions should begin to wilt. At
30 minutes, they'll take on a deep golden hue. That's

your cue to turn the heat back up. Allow the onions to stick slightly to the pan and deglaze with $^1/_2$ cup of liquid. Stir with a wooden spoon until all the liquid has evaporated.

Deglazing

This refers to adding liquid and scraping up the bits of food that are stuck to the bottom of the sauté pan (that stickiness is the food's sugar, which is outrageously delicious!). The pan may look like you have overcooked the food, but that's not the case. Just add a little liquid (wine, broth, or water) and quickly move the food around with a spoon or spatula to loosen all those flavorful bits. This also makes cleaning the pan a breeze.

FASS

A system of making dishes taste their best by balancing their flavors. FASS stands for fat, acid, salty, and sweet. This method utilizes simple, healthy ingredients such as extra virgin olive oil (fat), fresh lemons and limes (acid), sea salt (salt), and Grade B organic maple syrup (sweet) to enhance taste and correct dishes that have gone awry. For a full explanation, see chapter 1.

Flavor Seal

A method for locking in the flavor of a prepared dish. An example is adding herbs and deglazing a pan to seal in the flavor of an onion or shallot that has been sautéed to a golden brown.

Parsley "Haircut"

To quickly remove stems from parsley or cilantro, hold a clean, dry bunch of parsley or cilantro at a downward 45° angle with your noncutting hand, with the "head" of the herb touching the cutting board. Use short, blunt angled strokes with the side of your chef's knife to scrape the herb and separate the leaves from stems.

Peeling (vegetables)

Besides the usual culprits (carrots, potatoes, and onions), I also peel celery and asparagus with a vegetable peeler, making it sweeter, less stringy, and easier to digest.

Poaching

Gentle cooking in liquid. The liquid should be just below the boiling point, with its surface barely quivering. This method produces a delicate flavor by infusing the flavor of the liquid into the food.

Puréeing

Using a food processor or your Vita-Mix high-speed blender to turn fruits and vegetables into an ultrasmooth, creamy consistency. For that silky perfection, be patient; you'll see and taste the difference!

Raking

We use this technique to keep rice and grains from sticking together. Raking helps dry the food after it cooks and prepares it for the next step in a recipe. As the name implies, raking should be done with a fork, not a spoon. A spoon promotes pasty rice.

Reduction

Rapidly boiling a liquid (usually stock, wine, or a sauce) until evaporation reduces its volume. The result is a thicker consistency and intensified flavors.

Roasting (meats and vegetables)

Oven-cooking food in an uncovered pan. This creates a well-browned exterior and moist interior. It is an excellent method for releasing a lot of flavor.

Roasting and Toasting (nuts and seeds)

This process releases the nuts' natural oils and increases their flavor. Roast nuts at 325°F (350°F for almonds) on a sheet pan. The roasting time depends upon the type and quantity of nuts. Roast almonds for 10 to 15 minutes, pistachios for 8 to 10 minutes, pecans for 7 to 8 minutes, and pine nuts for only 2 to 4 minutes (don't walk away . . . they burn quickly!). Roast a lot at one time, some to eat and some to freeze. To toast, place seeds in a small frying pan over medium heat. Don't walk away from the stove or your seeds will be toast—not toasted. Shake the pan over the heat until the seeds become fragrant, about 3 minutes.

Sautéing
To cook food rapidly in a small amount of oil.

Slurry
A thin paste made with cold water and a thickening agent such as kudzu, arrowroot, or cornstarch. The paste is then whisked into a simmering sauce, soup, or stew.

Soaking (grains and rice)
This process breaks down the whole grain acids, improving our ability to digest and absorb nutritional benefits, especially B-complex vitamins. Soak grains overnight (or for at least 8 hours) in a bowl by covering them with warm water and the juice from half a lemon.

Spa Treatment (for canned and frozen vegetables)
Canned foods often lose some of their taste. Re-energize these foods, especially beans, by adding a spritz of lemon or lime juice and a pinch of salt. Frozen items get a spritz of lemon after defrosting.

Yum Factor
Finding that perfect taste balance that makes one's taste buds moan involuntarily with joy!

Zest
The outer rind of citrus fruits (usually oranges, lemons, or limes) used to enhance flavor. The best way to remove the zest is by raking a microplane grater across the fruit's surface. Before zesting, please thoroughly wash the fruit.

Resource Guide

THERE ARE HUNDREDS OF NUTRITIONAL, culinary, agricultural, and organic resources now available to consumers, especially those with access to the Internet. Here are a few, including a website that lists the farmers' markets closest to your home.

Food Resources
Whole Foods Market, the first certified organic supermarket: www.wholefoods.com

Organic Kitchen, a great one-stop organic cooking shop: www.organickitchen.com

Diamond Organics, for delivery nationwide of organic produce, groceries, and hard to find items: www.diamondorganics.com

Living Tree Community Foods, a source for organic oils, nuts, and nut butters: www.livingtree.com

Spectrum Organics, information on healthy cooking oils: www.spectrumorganics.com

Wilderness Family Naturals for coconut oil, milk, and more: www.wildernessnaturals.com

The Grain and Salt Society, information on salt and sea vegetables: www.celtic-seasalt.com

Maine Coast Sea Vegetables, a source for sea vegetables: www.seaveg.com

Rising Tide Sea Vegetables, for more on sea vegetables: www.loveseaweed.com

Maple Valley Syrups, for Grade B organic maple syrup: www.maplevalleysyrup.com

Lagier Ranches, for organic almonds sliced, whole, and everything in between: www.lagierranches.com

McFadden Farm, for organic herbs: www.mcfaddenfarm.com

Cascadian Farms, for frozen vegetables year-round: www.cfarm.com

Black Wing, a source for organic, free-range chicken: www.blackwing.com

Lundberg Farms, for information about rice products: www.lundberg.com

Crown Prince, canned salmon, sardines, and tuna made for the natural food industry: www.crownprince.com

Vital Choice, a source for wild line-caught salmon and other high quality seafood: www.vitalchoice.com

Eco Fish, a source for environmentally responsible seafood: www.ecofish.com

Eat Well Guide, a state-by-state listing of sustainably raised meats: www.eatwellguide.com

Bob's Red Mill, for a variety of flours, including gluten-free products and almond meal: www.bobsredmill.com

Arrowhead Mills, for organic and gluten-free grains and baking mixes: www.arrowheadmills.com

Summer's Sprouted Flour Company, for easy to digest organic sprouted wheat and spelt flours: www.creatingheaven.net/eeproducts/eesfc/

Kitchen Equipment Resources
Vita-Mix, the blender I use to purée everything: www.vitamix.com

Metro Kitchen: www.metrokitchen.com

Bridge Kitchenware: www.bridgekitchenware.com

cooking.com, everything for the household: www.cooking.com

Sur La Table: www.surlatable.com

Williams-Sonoma: www.williamsonoma.com

Farmers' Markets Resources
Local Harvest, for the best listings of farmers' markets, community supported agriculture (CSA) programs, and availability of organic produce in your area: www.localharvest.org

U.S. Department of Agriculture's Nationwide Farmers' Market Finder: www.ams.usda.gov/farmersmarkets/map.htm

Slow food, an international community of people devoted to preparing—and enjoying—food without rushing: www.slowfoodUSA.org

The Organic Center, for the latest science and news about organics: www.organic-center.org

The Organic Trade Association, for more information on organic foods: www.ota.com

Nutrition Resources
World's Healthiest Foods, for information on subjects related to nutrition and health: www.whfoods.com

U.S. Department of Agriculture's National Nutrient Database, for nutritional databases on every food from apples to zucchini: www.nal.usda.gov/fnic/foodcomp/search/

Resources for Living with Cancer
The National Cancer Institute: www.cancer.gov

Commonweal Cancer Help Program: www.commonweal.org

The Collaborative on Health and the Environment: www.cheforhealth.org

National Coalition for Cancer Survivorship: www.canceradvocacy.org

Association of Cancer Online Resources: www.acor.org

Appendix:
QUICK REFERENCE:
Preparation and Storage Time Chart

Recipes to Live For	Prepare Ahead	Prep Time	Cooking Time	Fridge Time	Freezer Time
All-Purpose Chicken Stock		15 minutes	2 hours	3 days	3 months
Almond Chocolate Chip Cookies	pulse almonds	15 minutes	1 hour	1 week	2 months
Anytime Crunch		15 minutes	1 hour		2 months
Asian Japonica Rice Salad with Edamame	make rice, roast nuts, dressing	30 minutes	1 hour	3 days	no
Asparagus Soup with Pistachio Cream	roast asparagus, magic mineral broth	1 hour	1 hour	2 days	3 months
Avocado Cream		30 minutes		1 day	no
Baby Bok Choy w/Sesame and Ginger	toast sesame seeds	30 minutes	10 minutes	2 days	no
Baby Dumpling Squash Stuffed with Rice Medley	roast squash, make rice	1 hour	1 hour	3 days	no
Best Oatmeal Ever	soak oats overnight	5 minutes	30 minutes	2 days	no
Black Bean Chili	Avocado Cream	30 minutes	30 minutes	3 days	3 months
Black Bean Medley	better made day before	1 hour		3 days	3 months
Bombay Beans	clean beans, store in fridge	30 minutes	30 minutes	3 days	no
Broccoli Sautéed with Garlic	blanch broccoli	15 minutes	15 minutes	1 day	no
Caramelized Sweet Red Onion Soup with Parmesan Crostini	caramelize onions or have premade in freezer	45 minutes	45 minutes	3 days	3 months
Carrot-Ginger Soup with Cashew Cream	cook carrots, sauté onions	30 minutes	30 minutes	3 days	3 months
Cashew Tart Crusts	bake and freeze unfilled	30 minutes	30 minutes	1 day	3 months
Chicken Patties with Apple and Arugula		1 hour	15 minutes	2 days	3 months
Chicken Potpie	chicken stock, pastry crust	1¹/₂ hours	45 minutes	3 days	3 months
Chicken . . . Roasted All the Way to Yum!		30 minutes	1 hour	3 days	1 month
Chicken Soup with Bowtie Pasta	chicken stock				no
Chicken Stew from My Nana	chicken, chicken stock				no
Chickpea Soup with Caramelized Fennel and Orange Zest	soak and cook beans ahead	1 hour	1 hour	3 days	3 months
Coconut-Ginger Rice with Cilantro	soak rice	15 minutes	45 minutes	3 days	no
Cornmeal Pizza	bake crust	45 minutes	30 minutes	3 days	1 month
Couscous Quinoa with Mint and Tomatoes		1¹/₂ hours		3 days	no
Dark Leafy Greens with Caramelized Onions, Raisins, and Pine Nuts	caramelize onions, toast pine nuts	30 minutes	15 minutes	2 days	no

Recipes to Live For	Prepare Ahead	Prep Time	Cooking Time	Fridge Time	Freezer Time
Delicata Squash with Dino Kale and Cranberries	roast squash	1 hour	1 hour	3 days	3 months
Emerald City Soup	Magic Mineral Broth	1 hour	1 hour	1 day	no
Flourless Almond Torte		30 minutes	30 minutes	3 days	3 months
Frittata with Herby Potatoes	roast potatoes	30 minutes	30 minutes	3 days	no
Fruit Compote	soak overnight	30 minutes	1½ hours	1 week	3 months
Fruit Crisp	make Anytime Crunch	15 minutes	1 hour	3 days	no
Fruit Parfait with Almond-Peach-Ginger Cream		1 hour	15 minutes	3 days	no
Garlicky Leafy Greens	wash and destem greens	30 minutes	15 minutes	3 days	no
Ginger Ale/Ginger Tea	freeze grapes, steep tea	5 minutes		1 week	
Gingerbread		30 minutes	45 minutes	3 days	1 month
Grandma Nora's Salsa Verde		5 minutes		1 week	3 months
Grape cubes		5 minutes			3 months
Herbed "Ricotta"	prepare tofu	1½ hours		3 days	3 months
Jicama and Red Cabbage Salad with Mint and Cilantro	cut vegetables, toast nuts, make dressing	1 hour		2 days	no
Kabocha and Butternut Squash Soup with Asian Pear, Apple, and Ginger	roast squash, Magic Mineral Broth	1 hour	1 hour	3 days	3 months
Kneadless Dough	make and freeze	5 minutes	15 minutes	2 days	1 month
Legal Cookies		30 minutes	1 hour	4 days	1 month
Lemon Caper Vinaigrette		10 minutes		1 week	no
Lemon Cashew Cream		10 minutes		3 days	no
Lemony Chicken with Capers and Kalamata Olives	marinate chicken	30 minutes	1 hour	2 days	1 month
Lemony Lentil Soup with Pistachio Mint Pesto	Magic Mineral Broth	1 hour	1 hour	3 days	3 months
Magic Mineral Broth		5 minutes	2½ hours	3 days	6 months
Miso-Ginger Soup with Udon Noodles		30 minutes	1 hour	3 days	no
Miso Salmon with Lime-Ginger Glaze	marinate salmon	30 minutes	30 minutes	1 day	no
Mixed Greens with Roasted Beets and Avocado	prep greens, roast beets, make dressing and pita crisps	2 hours		1 day	no
My Favorite Salad	make dressing	30 minutes	10 minutes		no
Orange Shallot Vinaigrette		1 hour		5 days	no
Pantry Pasta	rinse beans	15 minutes	10 minutes	2 days	no
Pestos		15 minutes		1 week	3 months

continues

Preparation and Storage Time Chart, *continued*

Recipes to Live For	Prepare Ahead	Prep Time	Cooking Time	Fridge Time	Freezer Time
Pita Crisps with Parmesan		30 minutes	15 minutes		no
Poached Coconut Ginger Salmon	coconut broth	2 hours	1 hour	1 day	no
Potato Comfort	cut potatoes and root vegetables	15 minutes	30 minutes	2 days	no
Puttanesca Sauce	roast tomatoes	1 hour	15 minutes	3 days	3 months
Salsa Variations		15 minutes		3 days	no
Sea-ser Dressing		15 minutes		1 week	no
Seasonal Couscous	roast squash	30 minutes	30 minutes	3 days	no
Smoothies		15 minutes		3 days	no
Spiced Roasted Almonds		5 minutes	15 minutes		6 months
Spinach Orzo with Pine Nuts and Feta	toast nuts	15 minutes	10 minutes	1 day	no
Stacked Polenta Pie with Garlicky Greens and Puttanesca Sauce	sauce and greens	15 minutes	30 minutes	2 days	no
Stir-Fry Sauce with Vegetables	slice vegetables	30 minutes	just minutes	1 week	no
String Beans with Caramelized Shallot, Rosemary, and Garlic	prep beans	1 hour	15 minutes	3 days	no
String Beans with Cherry Tomatoes and Feta Cheese	clean beans	30 minutes	15 minutes	2 days	no
Swiss Chard Braised with Sweet Tomatoes and Corn	wash chard	45 minutes	15 minutes	2 days	no
Swiss Chard Pasta		20 minutes	30 minutes	2 days	no
Swiss Chard "Ricotta" Gallettes	prepare Swiss chard, "Ricotta"	1 hour	1 hour	3 days	3 months
Szechwan Broccoli	blanch broccoli	30 minutes	15 minutes	1 day	no
Taxicab Yellow Tomato Soup with Fresh Basil Pesto	roast tomatoes, Magic Mineral Broth	1 hour	1 hour	3 days	3 months
Tortilla Stack with Salsa Cruda	prepare salsa	1 hour	15 minutes		no
Turkey Patties		1 hour	15 minutes	2 days	3 months
Tuscan Bean Soup with Kale	soak and cook beans, Magic Mineral Broth	1 hour	1 hour	3 days	3 months
Veggie "Ricotta" Lasagna	prepare greens, Herbed "Ricotta"	2 hours	1 hour	3 days	3 months
Yukon Gold Potato Leek Soup	Magic Mineral Broth	1 hour	1 hour	3 days	3 months

Index